The Secrets of Health

=

The Secrets of Wealth

A Chance to Live More Than 100 Years

Rich Finegan

To my daughter, Carisha Machiko, my son, Kenji Finegan, and my wife, Elita Tjandra, who used to be complained by me for sleeping earlier and waking up later than me; but now I know that she is right. I wish to be with her for more than 100 years in a healthy and wealthy life.

- 0 -

Table of Contents

- 0 -

The Introduction

- 0 -

Chapter 1

Introduction

Son   : *Mom!! There is an ant!!*

Mom   : *Where is the ant? Mmm...It is just a small animal.*

Son   : *But...but I am afraid that it will bite me.*

Mom   : *Don't worry. The ant is a small animal, and your body is bigger than an ant. What are you afraid of? Take your breath and blow on the ant, and it will go away!*

Son   : *Yes, Mom, It went away now. I am not afraid of ants anymore.*

Mom   : *Hattchiii...! (Sneezing)*

Son   : *Are you sick, Mom?*

Mom   : *Yeah, Mom has the flu.*

Son   : *Mom, what caused flu?*

Mom   : *Flu is caused by virus, which is like a small animal, much smaller than an ant. You cannot see it.*

Son   : *Mom, you said a virus is smaller than an ant, so what are you afraid of? Just blow it out of your body, Mom!*

Mom   : *You are right, son! Mom will blow it out of mom's body. Mom is not afraid of viruses anymore.*

That simple conversation will make you realize that a virus or bacterium is smaller than an ant; you are bigger and stronger than they are. Just blow them out, and they will go away.

If you are in sick, you can use your imagination to blow all the viruses and bacteria out of your infected body. I hope you are getting better before reading the next chapter.

Try this five-minute imagining—one hour after a meal:
Take deep, slow breaths through your nose, and then, with your eyes closed, slowly blow all the viruses and bacteria out of your body through your mouth. Focus on your mind.

Once you have an image of blowing the viruses or bacteria, your energy and spirits are there to heal your body. Don't underestimate this way of healing because it can restore your spirit or heal you—even wake you up from bed.

However this thought-based way of healing can't last long without a good immune system in your body. You can repeatedly have the flu or another disease if your immune system is weak. Then you should start from zero again. It is just like a cockroach in your house that always returns, even when you think you have exterminated all of them. Why do they return? Because they like your house's environment. This also happen when the virus or bacteria likes your body's environment—it will come again.

Other than viruses and bacteria, there are other diseases that are caused by body metabolism [1] problems, such as abnormal cells, stroke, high blood pressure, liver disease, kidney disease, etc.

Body metabolism problems sometimes are not easy to handle because they are more on people eating and living habits. There are thousands of health books published in this world and thousands of doctors who specialize in nutrition available but there are still many people who get sick because of these problems; people read health books and listen to doctors' advice but do not follow them consistently because:

- The health books and doctors want to change people's eating habits.
- People don't like to eat the recommended foods.
- The recommended foods are not readily available.
- The recommended foods are expensive.

What if a doctor advises you to avoid milk or cheese? You probably argue that you drink milk every morning, and there are millions of healthy people who drink milk or eat cheese daily. You can find lots of reasons to reject the advice because you think that the doctor wants to change your daily eating habits or the doctor wants you to give up your favorite foods. Ultimately, you get bored with their diet programs.

This book does not give you any recommendation on the foods you should or should not eat; you can still eat your daily

---

[1] Body Metabolism: all the physical and chemical processes in the body that create and use energy (i.e. digesting, blood circulation, excretion, function of brain, etc)

foods/meals but with certain conditions, so you can have a healthy life. You make the decision to lead a healthy life after learning the secrets of healthy living.

After reading this book you will understand that there is no food for longevity in this world. Just because the world's oldest person drinks green tea doesn't mean you must follow him. The food you currently eat can also make you healthy because you are not just what you eat; there are other important factors that can increase your health and give you a chance to live more than 100 years.

After many years of research and observation, I found that the secrets of health are the same as the secrets of wealth. If people in this world can be wealthy, they can be healthy too because both wealth and health have the same formula.

This book is divided into four parts; part one is the introduction of the concept that explains the basic information behind the concept; part two is the concept of this book; part three is the summary of important points, jokes, and frequently asked questions regarding to the concept; and part four is the appendix.

Chapter 2

Temperature around Us

A. Internal temperature

Before we were born into this world, we stayed in our mother's womb to develop body organs and cells during nine months. That place is not too hot or cold, and the temperature is around 36° to 37°Celsius (96.8° to 98.6° Fahrenheit). We can call this temperature range **warm temperature**.

If we are born sick or premature, a doctor will place us in an incubator with that warm temperature, so we can recover soon. The reason for using an incubator is to make the ambient temperature the same as the temperature of your mother's womb, so we will not waste our energy trying to adapt to outside temperature; instead, our energy is used for developing, healing, and growing our body. When we were a baby, we derived our energy mainly from milk, and the milk was prepared at warm temperature to avoid stomach problems such as flatulence (gas in our stomach).

With all these facts, we can say that in the beginning of our life, our bodies maintain a temperature of 36° to 37° Celsius (96.8°

to 98.6° Fahrenheit), and this temperature is our normal body temperature.

Why is it so important to know this internal temperature? Because when we are sick, our body condition may be as weak as a newborn baby, and we need to save our energy for useful things. By knowing our normal body temperature, we can use that temperature as a standard to cure or heal any diseases in our body and to increase our immune system.

How hot is our normal body temperature? You can touch your finger to your saliva or tongue or you can blow hot air from your mouth slowly to your hand, it won't burn your skin.

If you stay in a room at this temperature around ten minutes, you may feel hot, uncomfortable, and start sweating; however If you drink water at this temperature, it will feel more comfortable than your current drinking water because that temperature is similar to your saliva temperature, and so far you've never complained about your saliva temperature, right?

B. External temperature

Once we are born into this world, we need to adapt to the external temperature such as room, weather, water we drink and use, food we eat, floor where we stand, etc. Our body also needs to release energy to adjust to differences in temperature between our body and those external temperatures.

There are two kinds of external temperatures:

a. Temperature of touchable things

The examples of touchable things' temperature are:

- Temperature of water for bathing, swimming, and drinking
- Temperature of the foods we eat
- Temperature of the floors on which we stand

If those touchable things are at our body temperature, we will feel more comfortable. Any temperatures above or below this temperature will cause a higher energy loss from our body.

b. Temperature of untouchable things

The examples of untouchable things' temperature are:

- Weather temperature
- Room temperature or air temperature

We don't need to live at our body temperature because we have skin and fats that can help our body maintain its temperature.

Research on Basal Metabolic Rate or BMR (the minimum calories or energy required to sustain life in a resting individual) discovered that the minimum energy lost from our body caused by external temperature is at 26° Celsius (78.8° Fahrenheit); so we can say that the untouchable things temperature above or below 26° Celsius (78.8° Fahrenheit) will cause a higher energy loss from our body.

From those two external temperatures, we can summarize:

a. We need to drink water or eat foods as close as our body temperature.

b. We need to adjust our room temperature as close as 26° Celsius (78.8° Fahrenheit).

Why do we apply two kinds of temperatures for our body?

In addition to having skin and fats in our body, there is a **heat conduction factor**, which is a flow of heat through a substance or material.

For example:

- We have two spoons, one is made of metal and the other is made of plastic; if we put those spoons into a glass of hot water for a few minutes, which spoon is hotter? Yes, the metal spoon. Why? Because metal is a better conductor of heat than plastic.

- We feel cooler if we're standing on ceramic floors than when we feel the air temperature in the room because ceramic floors are better conductors than air.

- We feel cooler when we touch water that is 26° Celsius (78.8° Fahrenheit) than we do staying in a room that temperature, because water is a good conductor and air is a bad conductor. We also feel cooler when we swim in a swimming pool with water that is 26° Celsius (78.8° Fahrenheit) than sitting beside the pool when the air is that temperature.

Now we know one of the reasons for applying two kinds of temperature for our body: air is bad conductor and water is good conductor.

Chapter 3

How We Can Get Sick

We can get sick because of viruses and bacteria [2] and body metabolism problem. They can make us sick when our body does not have enough energy to fight or fix all those things.

Our energy is used for producing our immune system, but viruses and bacteria are always trying to take our energy, make us weak, or block the energy supply to our body cells and nerves. Once we run out of energy, they will stay in our body and become a disease.

We can eat three times a day, have healthy foods and drinks, and exercise regularly, but there is no guarantee that we can't get sick. There may be something stealing our energy, and we may never realize it.

What/who is stealing our energy? **ENVIRONMENTS**

---

[2] Viruses and bacteria are germs; there are other germs called fungi and protozoa. Viruses and bacteria are used in this book to simplify explanations.

Yes, environments steal our energy, make our body weak, and unprepared for attack by viruses or bacteria; even harmless viruses or bacteria that are exist in our body can threaten our life.

There are two kinds of environments that can take our energy:

1. External environment

This is the external temperature such as cold or hot weather, cold or hot room temperature, cold or hot drinking water, etc.

In cold weather people tend to get influenza and in hot weather people tend to get cough; this is because body energy is released to adapt to the weather temperature. Having influenza or cough can be an indication that our energy is getting weaker and cannot produce enough antibodies to fight the viruses.

In modern world, most people find it difficult to live without an **air conditioner (AC)**. The AC can be in bedrooms, office rooms, hotels, shopping malls, hospitals, toilets, cars, trains, etc. The invention of the refrigerator makes our life more fun, however with all these new inventions (AC and the refrigerator), we are actually far from our natural body temperature.

The worst thing from the external environment is**: we drink water at AC temperature or refrigerator temperature**. We unconsciously put a glass or drinking jar in our room (office, car, hospital, etc.) where the AC temperature is 15° to 25° Celsius (59° to 77° Fahrenheit), while our body temperature is 36° to 37° Celsius or 96.8°-98.6° Fahrenheit; there is a temperature shock in our stomach when we drink that cold water.

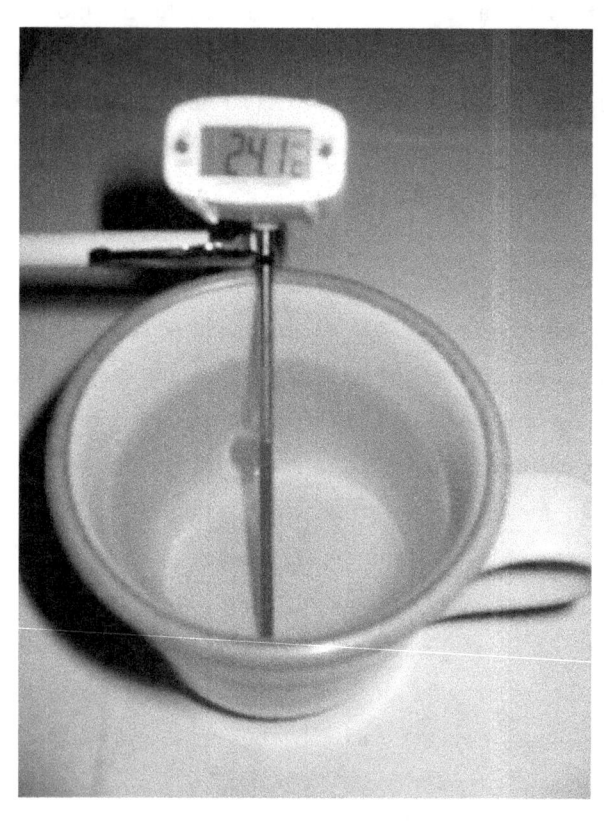

(Cold drinking water at 24.1° Celsius in an AC room)

Drinking water from a refrigerator or drinking water with ice (around 10° Celsius or 50° Fahrenheit) can give our stomach an even bigger temperature shock. It is similar to having somebody pour ice water on your face when you are sleeping. You will be shocked, and very angry with that person.

Temperature shock is a condition when our body encounters external things or environments that have a different temperature from our body and some of the body's energy is released to adjust to that difference.

Temperature shock is caused by drinking cold (or hot) water regularly. It may cause stomach or digestion problems because our stomach instantly produces stomach acid to accommodate that cold water, but there's no food to digest. This may cause the sudden death of some cells in our stomach or some digestive enzymes won't be able to work properly and spoil. You can try this by drinking cold water from a refrigerator and letting the cold water stay in your mouth for five second and then eating cookies. You will have a different taste and feeling in your mouth if you drink warm water and then eat the cookies. This means the enzymes in your mouth and your nerves were affected by a temperature shock.

Our dentist always advises us not to ingest food or drinks that are too cold or too hot because the temperature extremes could cause problems with our teeth in the future. The dentist never specifies the criteria for too hot or cold; now we know that too cold or hot is measured against our body temperature. Any foods or drinks which are higher or lower than 36° to 37° Celsius

(96.8° to 98.6° Fahrenheit) can cause a shock to our mouth, teeth, and stomach. It can be a big shock or a small shock; of course 10° Celsius (50° Fahrenheit) will have a bigger shock than 28° Celsius (82.4° Fahrenheit) or 50° Celsius (122° Fahrenheit) will have bigger shock than 40° Celsius (104° Fahrenheit).

Another example of temperature shock is walking without sandals or shoes or socks in a hospital room or in your house (bedroom, living room, etc) when the floor temperature is as cold as AC temperature. Your body energy will be stolen by that cold floor through your feet.

How many calories are wasted by a temperature shock?
There is formula to calculate the calorie loss caused by drinking water:

> Heat = Mass (grams) x (Temperature 2 – Temperature 1) Celsius

For example:
- We have two liters (2000 grams) of water at 23° Celsius (80.6° Fahrenheit), and we want to warm it to 37° Celsius (98.6° Fahrenheit); how many calories (energy) are used to warm that water?

    Answer:

    Heat = 2,000 grams x (37°-23°) Celsius

    = 2,000 x 14 = 28,000 calories or **28 Kcal**

People normally need around 2,000 Kcal to 3,000 Kcal (average 2,500 Kcal) in a day; however with more activities, some people may need more than 3,000 Kcal. Given these energy needs, it would seem that the impact of the energy loss from drinking that cold water is quite small—around 1 percent of energy lost (28 Kcal/2500 Kcal).

Let's look at several arguments on the important values of 1 percent energy loss:

- It takes more than twelve hours plus sleeping activity to convert energy from foods to body energy and distribute it to the body's cells.

- Not 100 percent of energy from foods is converted to body energy, and that means energy is lost during the process.

- The generated energy is used for keeping the function of heart, lungs, kidneys, digestive systems, and body temperature. There are many allocations of energy to body organs. If the energy allocation for our stomach is around 5 percent to 10 percent (assume average 7.5 percent), that means 1 percent of energy lost is equal to 15 percent of energy allocated to our stomach (28 Kcal/ (7.5%x2,500 Kcal))

- Our digestive enzymes work well at body temperature, and if we drink cold water (or hot water), it means those enzymes cannot work properly and will spoil, and our body will need more energy to produce those enzymes again.

- Doctor's advice: don't give too much cold drinking water to a baby because it may cause stomach problems, i.e., flatulence (gas in stomach) and eating problems.
- When people are sick and have a fever, they tend to drink warm water to save their energy.

In summary, don't underestimate the effect of 1 percent energy loss from our body or around 15 percent energy loss from the stomach because it affects many things in the overall food-energy process. The point is not to determine the exact percentage of lost energy from our stomach (I believe it is difficult to find the exact amount), rather it is that there is an energy loss in part of our energy generator systems. This is different from losing energy through your skin or other activities. (You may check with an engineer about how important 1 percent or 1 millimeter variance in a nuclear energy generator system is.)

There is a chaos theory in mathematics called the **butterfly effect** that states that small variations of the initial condition of a dynamical system may produce large variations in the long-term behavior of the system. An example of this theory is a butterfly flapping its wings in Africa can affect the weather in New York, United States of America.

The loss energy from the stomach before it digests foods can also mean unpredictable and unexpected results for the body over time, including stomachache, anemia, abnormal cells, high cholesterol, heart attack, kidney disease, liver disease, or other metabolism problems.

Simple explanation: If a cake needs warm water to mix all the ingredients, but we use cold water, the resulting cake may have a taste, texture, or color that we may not want. We may start grumbling. This is like the digestive system when the body needs warm water (body temperature) to mix and process all the foods with enzymes in stomach, but we ingest cold water. The result may not what our body wants, it may start grumbling, and we may develop metabolism problems over time.

Our energy is similar to our money

We work hard for money, and usually we won't let other people steal our money. Our energy is similar to money: we buy and eat foods for energy, and we should not let environments steal our energy. Money is to protect us from the cruel and hard environments in our daily life. Energy is to protect us from the cruel and hard environments in our body such as viruses, bacteria, abnormal cells, body metabolism problems, etc.

With money, we can ask people to kill cockroaches; with energy, we can also ask our immune system to kill the viruses and bacteria or to fix the abnormal cells in our body.

Here is the list of external environments that can waste our energy in daily life; we should be aware of the need to control them.

External environment that can waste our energy
Cold & Hot drinking water
Cold & Hot water for bathing
Cold & Hot floors
Cold & Hot room temperature
Cold & Hot weather

2. Internal Environment

Your internal environment includes your negative emotions such as: anger, sadness, jealousy, fear, panic, nervousness, shock, worry, frustration, anxiety, depression, and stress.

These negative emotions can take most of our energy if we can't handle it; no matter how many healthy foods we eat and how much exercise we take, we can fall sick because of this environment.

Internal environment (negative emotions) can be more destructive than external environment; it takes only a few days to make you sick. Your situation will be worse if those negative emotions create sleeping problems for you because you won't be able to recover your lost energy. Also, your organs such as liver, kidneys, heart, lungs, and digestive organs can be hurt by these emotions, so make sure you have enough good sleep when you are heavily affected by those emotions.

Internal Environment that can waste our energy (Negative emotions)			
Anger	Fear	Shock	Anxiety
Sadness	Panic	Worry	Depression
Stress	Nervousness	Frustration	Jealousy

Chapter 4

How to Control Environments

Realizing that our energy is similar to money, we know we need to save and protect it from environments; we can't eliminate those environments, but we can control them, so their impact on the body will be minimal.

A. External Environment:

In chapter 2 we discussed temperature around us, and we mentioned that the best touchable things temperature (water, foods, floors, etc) for our body is 36° to 37° Celsius (96.8° to 98.6° Fahrenheit), and the best untouchable things temperature (weather, room temperature) for our body is 26° Celsius (78.8° Fahrenheit). Using this information, we can do several things to control environments for our health benefits such as:

1. Take sweat bathing

Increase room temperature by using a room heater to 36° to 37° Celsius (96.8° to 98.6° Fahrenheit); if a room heater is not available, we can turn off the air conditioner and wear necessary clothes but make sure the room has enough air circulation by closing the door or windows halfway. We can sit, walk, or lay in the room watching TV or reading for about ten minutes to one hour. We can have a sweat bath once or twice in a week, depending on body condition.

After sweat bathing, try to adjust slowly from that hot room temperature to normal temperature (e.g., open the door/windows slowly or adjust the heater or AC slowly) to avoid sudden temperature shock in the body.

The benefit of sweat bathing:

- It removes toxins from our body.
- It increases our blood circulation.
- It reduces the kidneys' work in cleaning waste from our blood.

This sweat bathing is similar to a baby incubator; as there is no adult incubator at the moment, but we can use a bedroom, car, tent, or other sauna room at warm temperature for sweat bathing. (You need to consider the smell from your sweat too.)

We do not use a common sauna (commercial sauna) for sweat bathing because common sauna room temperature is usually around 60° to 100° Celsius (140° to 212° Fahrenheit).

Notes:

For the first time, we can start room temperature at 30° Celsius (86° Fahrenheit) and increase it slowly to 37° Celsius (98.6° Fahrenheit), after several days or weeks of exercises. If we can sweat at 30° Celsius (86° Fahrenheit), let's use this temperature for our sweat bathing standard, and it is not necessary to reach 37° Celsius (98.6° Fahrenheit). **The point is to sweat in a normal way and not exceed our body temperature.**

- If we exercise regularly, we don't have to do this sweat bathing because we regularly sweat in a normal way.
- This exercise is more applicable to those who seldom sweat, i.e., back office worker or those who have a physical disability.
- If you are in hospital or sick, please seek your doctor's advice before practicing sweat bathing.
- Sweat bathing can release our energy, but we release it for useful activity, and it is good for our health.

2. Always drink warm water

In our modern world, having stomach or digestive problems is common. People have tried without success to eliminate these problems by eating three meals daily on a schedule, eating healthy food, do not eat chili, and reducing stress. They do not realize the negative effect of drinking cold (iced) water or water at AC temperature on a daily basis.

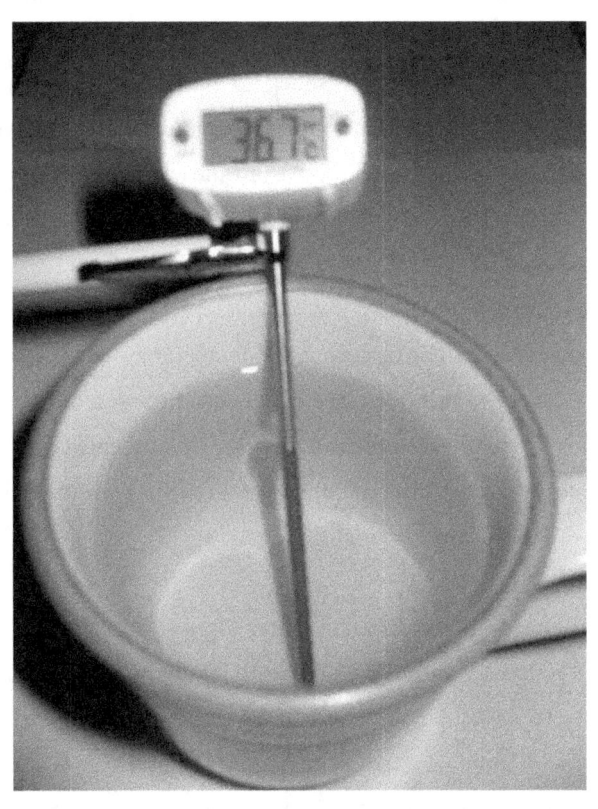

(Warm drinking water at 36.7° Celsius- healthy)

It is common for employees in the office or people who just wake up in the morning to drink cold water at AC-room temperature, and this cold water will cause temperature shock for their stomach.

To avoid temperature shock to the stomach, we need to make a daily habit of drinking warm water. Initially you will need a thermometer to measure the water's temperature to get a feel for 36° to 37° Celsius (96.8° to 98.6° Fahrenheit) temperature. After several days, your mouth will know automatically if the water is the proper temperature. We don't have to be perfect at that temperature level. **The point is to try to minimize the difference between our drinking water temperatures and our body temperature, so we do not waste additional energy and create high temperature shock for our stomach.**

3. Take a bath with warm water

Try to use warm water (around 36° to 37° Celsius or 96.8° to 98.6° Fahrenheit) for bathing, especially when we are in sick condition, tired, or taking a bath at night. Warm water can prevent temperature shock to our body.

4. Take sun bathing

A few minutes (five to ten minutes) in a day under the morning sun can also warm our body (we do not have to sweat). Some research also mentions that sun bathing can make several vitamins work well in our body, especially vitamin D, which is good for our heart, good for increasing our body's immunity, and regulating blood pressure.

5. Wear sandals or socks or shoes on a cold floor or hot floor.

This looks funny and uncommon, but those floors, and especially ceramic floors, will have a similar temperature with AC temperature in the room. Wearing sandals or socks or shoes can keep our feet warm, and this can prevent additional energy loss from our body.

6. Set room temperature as close to $26°$ Celsius ($78.8°$ Fahrenheit) as possible

As explained in chapter 2, our body will lose its minimum energy at external temperature $26°$ Celsius ($78.8°$ Fahrenheit); so it is a good idea to adjust our room temperature to that temperature. If that's not possible, we can try to adjust our clothes.

Offices, schools, hospitals, supermarkets typically have an ambient temperature of around 15° to 25° Celsius (59° to 77° Fahrenheit) because they need to consider the number of people inside their buildings and also the outside weather temperature.

For our bedroom, we can set auto AC temperature at $26°$ Celsius ($78.8°$ Fahrenheit); however, sometime we still feel hot or cold with that temperature setting because the outside weather temperature affects our room temperature. The best way is to look at our room thermometer and make the necessary AC temperature adjustments to make our room temperature as close to 26° Celsius (78.8° Fahrenheit) as possible.

7. Sleep for seven to eight hours a day

Sleeping is the process for restoring our energy. All the foods we eat can be absorbed well by our body's cells if we have enough sleep. Sleeping is the best way to keep our body warm. We will discuss more on sleeping in chapter 6 The Secret of Sleeping.

B. Internal Environment:

Handling internal environment is more difficult than external environment because it involves human emotions.

There are several ways to reduce our internal environment problems (negative emotions):

1. Take a slow, deep breath (in and out) for three to five minutes while closing the eyes

We don't need to imagine any positive emotions (happy, joyful, peaceful, forgiven, etc.), just let our breath wash out the negative emotions. We can sit or lie on the bed or stand up positions for this exercise.

2. Engage in light exercise such as walking for fifteen minutes outside our room.

By having this exercise, we are releasing energy for useful activity that can increase our health. Once we release this energy, our negative emotions can be reduced to lower our tension.

3. Go to sleep

Instead of wasting energy on negative emotions, it is better we go to sleep (save our energy) and forget all the problems.

Having a consultation with a doctor or psychologist is the best choice if the negative emotions disturb your sleep for several days. Don't save money for this consultation fee because your energy leakage may cost you more in the future.

Chapter 5

The Energy

The simple answer on how we can get sick is our body does not have enough **energy** to fight the viruses and bacteria or fix the body metabolism problems.

We now know that energy is the main issue in our health system, so let's find out what forms our energy.

Source of Energy

Our body energy comes from the food we eat, and to convert the food to energy for the body's use, we need another two external things that are more important than the food itself—air and water. So we can say that our body energy is formed by:

1. Air we breathe,

2. Water we drink, and

3. Food we eat.

Air we breathe

We can die if we do not breathe for a few minutes, so the quality of the air in our environment is very important. We can see that people who live in mountain areas look fresher and healthier than those living in the city. If you are assuming that those people do not have any life problems, you are not 100 percent right because everyone has problems, even in the mountains.

What do you feel when you are in a mountain area? Do you feel fresher and at peace? Besides the views, a mountain area has a lot of oxygen to boost your energy, and this fresh energy is strong enough to clear your negative emotions.

If your families or friends have problems that have caused high stress, depression, or even led to thoughts of suicide, you can ask them to go to mountain area for a few days before they want to leave this world. Mountain areas can give them more energy to think more clearly and solve their problem.

Water we drink

Water is more important than food because people can die faster without it (about three days) than eating (about one to two months). So the quality and amount of water you drink is more important than the quality and amount of food you eat.

Drinking warm water, which is similar to your saliva and body temperature, should be your first choice because it is the nature of our life

Food we eat

Each country has its own food; people in China may not eat the same food as people in Africa, Japan, India, Indonesia, or Switzerland. Even within a country, people who live in mountain area and a beach area have different kinds of food; with all these different kind of foods, each country has its very elderly people (more than 100 years). This means God is not really concerned about what you eat in this world, as long as the foods are not poisonous. We will discuss more about foods in chapter 7 Healthy Food and Balanced Eating.

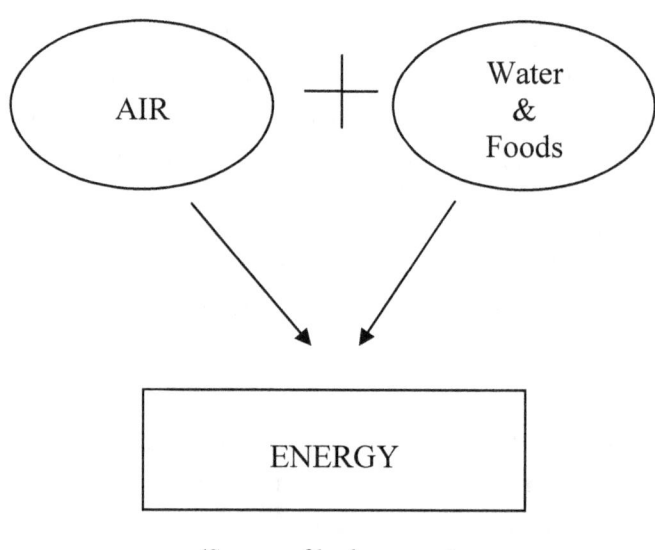

(Source of body energy)

Energy Distribution

The food energy in our body is distributed to body cells by blood flowing through blood vessels, and the regulator of this distribution is our **brain**.

To illustrate this, we can say that our brain is a war general, our body is a castle, and we are the king.

The war general duties are:

- To make sure all the military systems are working well,
- To make sure his soldiers have enough food and rest,
- To arrange strategy to defend the castle from inside and outside enemy attack.

With all those important tasks, of course the war general must get enough sleep, so he can concentrate and do his duties well. If that war general does not have enough sleep, he can't concentrate on his duties, his soldiers may not get enough food, all the military systems may not work well, and the soldiers are easily persuaded to betray the war general or the king. This will give the enemies chance to win the war, take over the castle, and then kill the king.

Similar to a war general, our brain needs sleep to make sure:

- All the functions of our body are working well, so there are no abnormal cells.
- All the body cells have enough energy and rest to defend our body from viruses and bacteria attack.

No matter how good the quality of the air, the water you drink, and the food you eat, if you do not have enough sleep, the generated energy cannot be distributed to and used by your body cells well.

Energy Expenditure

The energy from our food will be used for daily activities, keeping internal organs (lungs, heart, digestive organs, kidneys, etc.) running well, keeping body at warm temperature, keeping the immune system working well, etc. Sometimes we spend or use this energy having fun doing things like watching TV, chatting, browsing the Internet, having a party or pursuing hobbies (which make us forget the time). Spending energy is similar to spending money. It is fun when we go shopping—buying electronics, cars, bags, watches, etc. There's nothing wrong with spending money as long as it is within our buying limit, and if we're using credit cards, we're not spending beyond our ability to repay in full amount when it is due. Otherwise there will be penalty and interest charged to us. Similar to the energy, when we feel tired or it is time to sleep, we should not spend our energy beyond its limit. It is better to get some rest or go to sleep and avoid medicines or coffee or energy drinks that can boost our energy because we can fall sick (get the penalty).

The Concept

- 0 -

Chapter 6

The Secret of Sleeping

In modern life, people seldom sleep for eight hours a night. Why? Look at your environments: cable TV, Internet, restaurants, supermarkets, foreign exchange market, and other amazing diversions are available twenty-four hours a day. How can you miss such things by sleeping? What about your office workload or family problems? How can you sleep at 10:00 P.M. when you reach your house or apartment at 10:00 P.M.?

If you are given two choices by God, which one will you choose?
1. Having a lot of money but in poor health
2. Having little money but in good health

Of course all of you want a lot of money and good health, but there is no such choice at the moment; you are only given those two choices.

From those two choices, most people tend to choose having little money but in good health. The reason could be:

- Healthy is more valuable than Wealthy
- If I have a lot of money and poor health, most of my money will go for medical bills (if you do not have insurance policy),
- I cannot enjoy this world, cannot travel, enjoy food, or have fun with my family and friends.
- I don't want to spend the rest of my life in my bedroom.

It sounds like an easy answer, but look at your life; does your job or lifestyle leave you enough time to sleep eight hours a night? Do you need to find other job or change your lifestyle or prepare exit-plan strategy for other job to have enough time to sleep eight hours in a twenty-four-hour period? Can you make a decision on which options you will choose now?

Research on people reveals that the optimum amount of sleep for adults is seven to eight hours; I would say that people need to sleep eight hours a night or seven hours at night plus a one-hour afternoon nap, i.e., you fall asleep at 10:00 P.M. and wake up at 6:00 A.M. or you fall asleep at 11:00 P.M. and wake up at 6:00 A.M. plus a one-hour afternoon nap. It is better to have a regular sleeping and waking time because your body can set an automatic biological clock for you so that you feel sleepy at 10:00 P.M. and you wake up at 6:00 A.M.

Sleeping is not a favorite topic for many people; people can just say "sleeping is sleeping," and it doesn't need any explanation, but in fact most people get less than eight hours of sleep in a twenty-four-hour period.

Sleeping is more important than eating healthy foods because people can die faster from not sleeping (about three days) than eating (about one to two months). Sleeping will make your body in a restful condition, so all your body cells can absorb the energy generated from your food. While sleeping, your damaged cells or nerves are replaced or repaired. Your brain, which is the master of your body control, can also take a rest, so it can regulate and manage body metabolism, nerve systems, immune system, and other systems in your body.

You will be fresher, warmer, and stronger when you wake up in the morning after sleeping eight hours because your body's cells will have received energy. Your body's muscles and mind will have taken a rest, and your body is ready to defend itself from viruses, bacteria, abnormal cells, pollution, or food preservatives and flavorings for the whole day with its available energy.

This conversation may give you a better understanding:

Max is an employee of a software company, and Bos is his manager.

Bos : *Max, can you download a film from the Internet? We have paid for it.*

Max : *Yes, how long does it take to download the film?*

Bos : *It is around eight hours.*

Max : *WHAT!! Eight hours??*

Bos : *Yeah, it is a big file. When you download it, please make sure you reach eight hours, otherwise we won't have the whole film.*

Max : *(After five hours of downloading and talking to himself) I have a date with my girlfriend, so I'll leave this computer to work itself until eight hours is up. I'll come back again tomorrow morning.*

Bos : *(Tomorrow morning) Max, have you finished downloading the film?*

Max : *My apology, Bos. Yesterday I left the computer after five hours of downloading because I had an urgent appointment. Unfortunately, we had an electricity problem in the office, and all the files are not completely downloaded yet.*

Bos : *Okay, that's all right but please make sure you do it today!*

(After trying for a week, Max still cannot complete the downloading process because he doesn't have the discipline to do it for eight hours! There is always an excuse for leaving the office early; he thinks that his computer can do it for him automatically, but it cannot.)

Bos : *(One week later) Max, sorry to say that I have to cut your salary because you are not doing your job well; I'll give you another chance to fix your habits.*

Max : *Okay, I will do my best, Bos. I accept the salary cut.*

(Two weeks later, Max still cannot change his habits to complete the eight hours of downloading, which according to him it is a waste of time, useless, and very boring)

Bos   : *Max, you are fired. Today is your last day. It is your habits that forced me to make this decision. If you had followed my instructions, I would have given you a bonus, but it is impossible now.*

Let's look at Max's sleeping habits and what he will get:

Max is a religious person; he believes in God and made God as his boss in his life.

God   : *Max, Can you do me a favor? It is just a sleeping job.*

Max   : *Yes, how long does it take to sleep?*

God   : *Around eight hours.*

Max   : *WHAT!! Eight hours??*

God   : *Yeah, it is a big job. When you are sleeping, make sure you get eight hours, otherwise I cannot show my power.*

Max   : *(After five hours of sleep and talking to himself) I have a job to do. I'll leave my body to take care the remaining three hours of sleep. I'll continue sleeping tomorrow.*

God   : *(Tomorrow morning) Max, have you finished sleeping for eight hours?*

Max   : *My apology God, Yesterday I had an urgent meeting that I could not miss. I'll continue the eight hours of sleep tomorrow.*

God : *Okay, that's all right, but please make sure you do it!*

(After trying for a week, Max still cannot manage to sleep eight hours at night because he doesn't have any discipline. There is always an excuse for Max to wake up early, and he thinks that his body can handle all the sleep debt, but it cannot.)

God : *(One week later) Max, sorry to say that you now have liver and heart diseases because you haven't done your job well. I'll give you another chance to fix your habits.*

Max : *Okay, I will do my best, God. I accept these diseases.*

(Two weeks later, Max still cannot change his habit to sleep eight hours a night, which according to him is a waste of time, useless, and very boring)

God : *Max, today is your last day. You must leave this world tonight. Your habit forced me to make this decision. If you had followed my instructions, I would have given you a healthy life and a chance to live more than 100 years. That's history now.*

The benefits of sleeping for eight hours a day:

1. The food energy can be fully absorbed by body cells. This will give you a stronger immune system, which can protect you from viruses or bacteria or abnormal cells in your body,

2. You will have better digestive system because the damaged cells from previous digestive process will be replaced by the new ones,

3. You will have a better defecation (feces) by having enough sleep,
4. Your mind will be more relaxed and can solve problems with better decisions (i.e., when you are having family problems, I suggest you and your partner get eight hours of sleep for several days. Don't wake up or leave your bed until you reach eight hours. I hope you can think more clearly, solve the problems, and have peace in your family),
5. You can have a better control of your body, so you can avoid unnecessary accidents that are caused by lack of sleep. There are hundred thousand or maybe millions of accidents in this world that are caused by a lack of sleep.

In the modern world, there are many reasons people have to sleep for eight hours in a day, so they will have enough energy to protect their body from damage and disease:

a. Many food preservatives and flavorings are developed to satisfy our tongue,
b. Pesticides and hormones are used in the cultivation of vegetables and fruits,
c. Air and water pollution,
d. Daily negative emotions such as stress, anger, and depression take a lot of energy.
e. Weather or climate change that is caused by global warming,
f. New viruses or bacteria mutations,
g. Side effects of medicines.
h. Mobile phone radiation

What if you do not sleep eight hours in a day?

Sleeping less than eight hours in a day will cause sleep debt, and to better understand sleep debt, you can look at credit card debt or other debt conditions. If you have a credit card debt, you need to pay at least a minimum payment but there will be a penalty added to the balance; if you do not make a payment, a debt collector will knock your door, ready to seize your computer, your TV, your AC, your sofa, and you never know when they will come to seize your assets.

Sleep debt is much the same; you can pay it tomorrow or at the weekend, but there will be penalties—your performance, emotions, and immune system will be affected. If you do not pay this sleep debt, it will seize your liver, kidneys, heart, stomach, intestines, lungs, nerves, etc. You will never know when it will seriously affect your health. So, it is better not to incur sleep debts by paying them in full daily—by sleeping eight hours a day.

Financial Leverage vs. Sleep Leverage

Financial leverage is a way to use borrowed money (debt) to finance an investment or a project with the expectation of greater return on your investment. The example of financial leverage is buying a property by using a bank loan. You pay 20 percent as a down payment and the 80 percent is paid by the bank loan (financial leverage). Using financial leverage can make people richer and poorer; to use financial leverage, you need to calculate carefully the cost and benefit such as the interest rate, penalty, due date, return period, investment return, etc.

Sleep leverage is a way to use more time to do jobs or tasks or activities by reducing sleeping time. For example, you work until 1:00 A.M. and wake up at 6:00 A.M. to chase your work deadline or to complete your idea. Sleep leverage can make you richer because you do the jobs faster than others, but also it can make you poorer because you can fall sick or have an accident.

Financial leverage and sleep leverage have significant differences:

Financial leverage	Sleep leverage
Reward: richer	**Reward:** richer and promotion
Risk: losing assets and poorer	**Risk:** losing life, sick, accident
Due date: more than 1 years	**Due date:** a few days [3]
Cost: interest expense, penalty	**Cost:** liver, kidneys, heart, etc

Do not use a short-term debt to finance a long-term investment because the long-term investment return may not be able to repay that short-term debt. This advice is considered sound investment policy in the financial world. In the case of sleep, sleep leverage is a very short-term debt and should not be used for reaching your long-term career or future financial goal because the risk is very high. **If you said that you work hard until midnight and do not sleep eight hours a day because you want to have a successful life and better future, you are using the wrong leverage and risk you life before you get the reward.**

---

[3] People can die from not sleeping for three days.

If you start working at age twenty-years-old and retire at sixty-years-old, it means you will have spent (or invested) forty years working, with the aim of earning money. You should ask for at least 100 percent return for the time you invest, which is another forty years to enjoy your life. This means you are still able to enjoy your life at least up to 100-years-old after retiring. Using the wrong leverage in your life may reduce your investment return. This means you can get sick and have some disease by your fortieth, fiftieth or sixtieth year—a common situation judging by the typical hospital.

Sleep leverage or sleep debt should be used for **urgent matters** only and needs to be paid as soon as possible. You should not use this leverage many times in daily life because the risk is higher than the rewards.

Mathematic calculation for sleep debt - simplified

For example, you eat food 2,500 Kcal in a day; it is converted to 2,500 Kcal of body energy and distributed to body cells by sleeping for eight hours a day. If you sleep for six hours in a day, part of the energy is not distributed well and wasted as body heat. Total wasted energy is (8-6)/8 x 2,500 Kcal = 625 Kcal, which is **a quarter of your energy from food**.

We can conclude:

- If you sleep for eight hours a day, you do not waste a quarter of your energy, and you can start reducing your meal for a quarter too (breakfast, lunch, and dinner), so the net energy is still the same.

- Sleeping for eight hours will maximize the absorption of food energy by your body cells.
- Sleeping for eight hours will help your digestive organs work well because you can eat less.

Simplified calculation for sleep debt:

Sleeping 6 hours in a day	Sleeping 8 hours in a day
Eat : 2,500 Kcal Wasted : 625 Kcal Net energy : 1,875 Kcal	Eat : 1,875 Kcal Wasted : 0 Kcal Net energy : 1,875 Kcal
Eat more, wasted some energy, net energy is 1,875 Kcal	Eat less , wasted zero energy, net energy is 1,875 Kcal – better digestion process

Sleeping Problem

Some people may have a sleeping problem, and it can be caused by stress, depression, jet lag, irregular sleeping time, hormone problem, or other disturbances such as noisy cars, fabrics, and neighborhood noise levels. However, as we know the benefit of sleeping, we need to find ways to solve these problems.

Here is an exercise that may solve your sleeping problem:
Lie on the bed and take long, regular breaths, do not think about anything; if this does not work, still in the long regular breathing, you can imagine a happy time in the past with your spouse or

children, or friends or any situation that makes you happy, smile and relax (i.e., first date with your spouse, first birthday of your child, funny thing you made when you were at senior high school or university).

If you are worried about your children, your wealth, or anything that belongs to you and this causes a sleeping problem for you, here is advice from a great wise man (Buddha):

The fool worries, thinking, "I have sons, I have wealth." Indeed, when <u>he himself is not his own</u>, whence are sons, whence is wealth? (Dhammapada 6:62)

When you are sick, you are alone, no one can help and feel your pain, so stop worrying anything when you are sleeping because you yourself are not your own.

The Secret of Sleeping

What are you doing when you have problems or wishes? Yes, praying!

Praying is communication with God or the universe, and to transmit your wish to God or the universe you should have enough energy to transmit it, otherwise God or the universe may not receive your wish clearly.

The transmission of a wish in prayer is similar to a transmission of a voice from a tape. If the tape does not have enough battery energy, you will have difficulty hearing the voice transmitted from the tape.

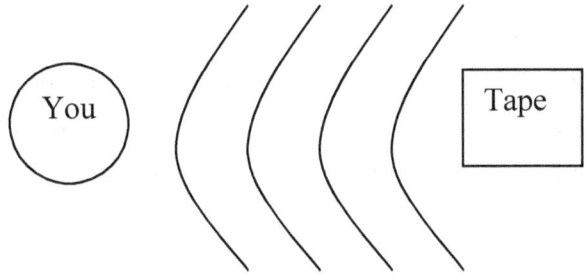

(A low battery tape transmission, the voice is not clear)

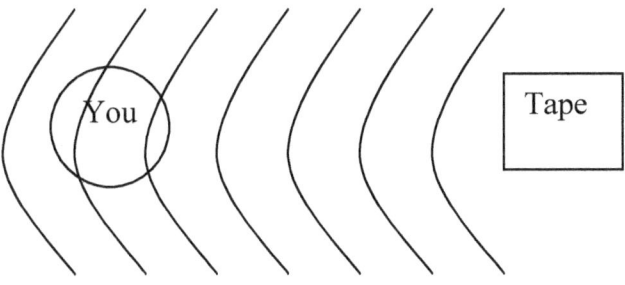

(A strong battery tape transmission, the voice is clear)

To have an effective prayer or wish, you need to have enough sleep for eight hours in a day, so you will have a strong energy (strong battery) to transmit your daily wishes to God or the universe. With strong energy, you can make wishes or make visualizations for your health, wealth, good family, good girl or boy friend, good careers, or any things in your dreams; because God has promised to give anything you want in your wishes (this is called the law of attraction, which is that what you think or visualize strongly is what you get in the future), so we can say that **sleeping for eight hours in a day is the secret of secrets in human life.**

The secret of secrets in human life both health and wealth

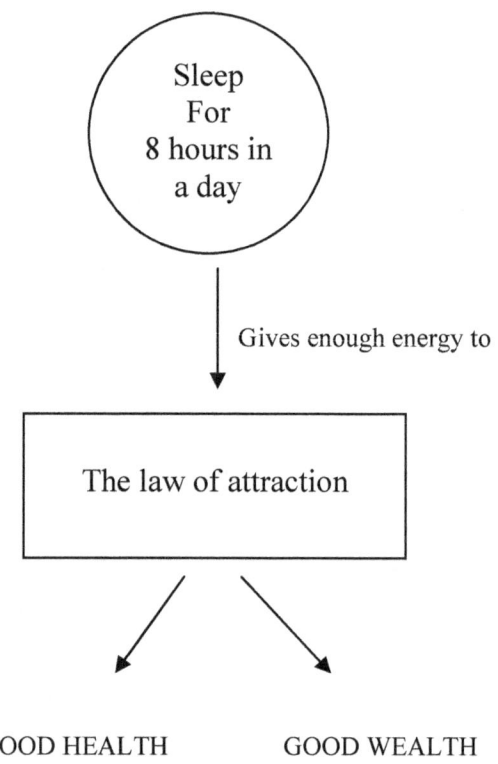

Chapter 7

Healthy Foods and Balanced Eating

In this chapter I want to share my views and make several comments about healthy foods and the health books around us; I do not make any recommendations on the foods you should or shouldn't eat because each of you may have different environments, daily activities, ages, and health conditions than me.

There are many health books written every day in this world, and we can find them easily in many bookstores; if you read several of them, you may get confused and not know what you should eat. Some books recommend that you eat based on blood type, but some may disagree and ask you not to take meats, eggs, milk, and cheese or even ask you to be a vegetarian. Most of those books are written by doctors or nutrition experts; it is hard to say that they are right or wrong because you may not have the knowledge to argue with them.

I have read many books on healthy foods, and to be honest, I used to be confused about which method is the best to follow. Some of those books are quite thick and too detailed; I couldn't remember what to eat or not to eat when I finished them. The most confusing thing is trying a method recommended in a best-selling health book, and then a few weeks later, a new health book is released that contradicts the method I've been following. What should I do—continue or stop or follow the new book's recommendation? Before answering this, let's look at this question first.

Do you need to change your meals according to the best-selling health book recommendations?

If your answer is: "*Yes, I need to change my meals according to the best-selling health book recommendations,*", you need to consider:

a. **Do you have a long-term commitment to follow the recommended foods?**

Within one to six months you may be able to follow the book recommendation, what about a commitment for one year, five years, or your whole life? You may find that your life is no longer fun because you cannot eat foods that you want to eat. Your restriction is coming from the book you read. You do not eat pizza because the book said that cheese and beef are not good for your health, but your little heart may have question why are people who are healthy still eating pizzas? Will they have shorter lives?"

b. **Are those recommended foods available in your living area?**

A healthy book may recommend that you eat fresh wheat, olive oil, certain fish or certain foods, but if you cannot find those foods in your area or country, you need to reconsider following that book recommendations.

c. **Are those recommended foods within your budget?**

Your health book may recommend that you eat imported foods that are quite expensive for your budget; you may need to reconsider this.

If your answer is: "*No, I don't need to change my meals according to the best-selling health book recommendation*"

You should think again because the writers are doctors or nutrition experts with many years of experience and observations; they can't be wrong 100 percent.

What you should do:

The best way is to have a consultation with a doctor or nutritionist in your city and discuss the foods suitable for your current health condition, age, environment, and activities.

You can also do basic research on what vegetables or fruits are planted within your locality. Vegetables or fruits that are planted nearby should be your first choice because those vegetables and fruits are planted in the similar environment, weather, and sunlight with your living area. Each vegetable and fruit has its own vitamin and mineral and nothing wrong for eating your local vegetables or fruits.

Some people said that grapes are good for health, but if your country does not produce grapes, it doesn't mean you won't be healthy by eating oranges or papayas. Wine is made from grapes, and it can be easily found in European countries. It may be good for people in those countries, but if you live in a country that has different weather, i.e., Africa, Arab countries, the wine may not be suitable for you.

You may also hear people say by eating an apple every day, you do not need a doctor. It is true that apples contain a lot of vitamins and minerals, but if your country does not produce this fruit, you don't have to worry. On the other hand, you should raise questions about this fruit; let's say the apples are from X country, and you are staying in Y country. How long does it takes the apples to be transported from the apple plantation to the warehouse for packing, to the destination warehouse or supermarket? Why are these fruits still fresh and shiny?

Don't Underestimate Your Body

If there is no health and religion constraint, foods that other people eat, you can also eat. (Of course, your body may need time to adjust to some new foods.) If you read health books and the authors ask you to avoid milk, eggs, meat, cheese, or other foods, you don't have to panic just because you eat those foods now. You can reduce the amount of those foods that you eat. For example, if you take seven eggs in a week, you can reduce that to three eggs in a week. Or if you drink milk every day, you can reduce it to three times in a week. Reducing all these foods can give your body more time to digest, absorb, or reject those foods from your body.

We just reduce the amount of those foods we eat and not avoid them (we do not follow 100 percent of the health books' recommendations) because you do not want to underestimate your body's ability to digest the foods, and also the authors may not be 100 percent right. There are several arguments for not following 100 percent health books recommendations:

- Their sample of observation can't represent the whole world with different kind of environments, activities, health conditions, ages, foods available, blood types, etc.

  For example:

  Do you agree with this survey conclusion?

  A survey to 400,000 people who subscribe XYZ magazine revealed that: 80 percent of married men tend to have secret affairs with their ex-girlfriends, and the conclusion is: 80 percent of married men in this world tend to have secret affairs with their ex-girlfriends.

  You agree because that survey involved 400,000 people, but what if a person said "It should be 80 percent of readers (men) of that XYZ magazine tend to have secret affairs with their ex-girlfriend, not the whole men in this world". Will that be a different view of survey conclusion?

- The main object for the observation is a group of older people, and then the authors may recommend you to take beans, wheat, and vegetables because most of those old people eat these kinds of foods. It is true that older people have slower body metabolism than younger people, and it is good to take mainly beans or wheat or vegetables for their meals and reduce intake of meats at their age. But it doesn't mean your kids or yourself have to be a vegetarian or only eat wheat, beans, and vegetables your whole life. Your age, environments, and foods available may be different from them.

- Sometimes the authors take the composition of a chimpanzee's diet as the basis for our diet. Humans are different from chimpanzees, our life and way of thinking are more complicated and complex, and we need more proteins and minerals from various kinds of foods to support our activities.
- You do not want to be sensitive or sick in the future because you avoid some foods now. For example, in a war or natural disaster or accident (earthquake, floods, shipwreck) there are not many foods available; you need to train your body enzymes to handle those foods once in a while but don't take it very often or too much.
- Each country has its own very old people and each of them eat different kinds of foods that are different from the authors' recommendations.
- Especially when you are allergic to the recommended foods, you do not have to follow the book's recommendations.

Food Composition

There are many foods compositions recommended by health books including World Health Organization (WHO); their recommendation can be 10 to 20 percent from protein, 20 to 30 percent from fats, and 50 to 65 percent from carbohydrates. The food composition is only a guide—there is no perfect diet.

Centuries ago, emperors sought the best foods and what to eat or avoid for longevity. We know that there is no food that guarantees longevity because food is not more important than a clean air, sleeping for eight hours in a day, and drinking warm water.

If the air is standard or the air pollution is acceptable, then sleeping for eight hours in a day and drinking warm water should be your priority for longevity not food compositions.

If you want to know some health books on food compositions, you can read **Hiromi Shinya's** *The Enzyme Factor*, several books written by **Dr. Peter J. D'Adamo** that include his recommendation on food based on blood types. You don't have to push yourself to find the food recommended in those books if they are not available in your area, just take notes on the foods you should reduce.

I believe that, in addition to Japan, there are many people near or more than 100 years old in China, India, Indonesia, Spain, and other countries. All the old people in different countries have their own food composition (don't have the same foods).

When to eat

People usually eat three times a day—around 7:00 A.M., 12:00 P.M. and 6:00 P.M.—because they are feeling hungry at those times. When the food reaches stomach, it will be digested and stay there up to four hours. That means that within four hours after your meal, it is better you do not eat anything except warm drinking water and fruits.

We drink warm water because all the enzymes in saliva and stomach are working well at warm temperature, and also we do not want to disturb the digested food temperature, which is either still in progress or nearing completion in our stomach.

If you drink cold water when the food is ready to be delivered to another part such as small intestine, liver, that cold water temperature will change the digested food (chyme) temperature to nonstandard temperature that will affect the food process. You may remember that water is a good conductor (chapter 2), so all the liquid material such as chyme, gastric acid, enzymes from stomach to intestines will be affected by this cold water temperature, and this may cause body metabolism and body immune system problems in the long term (this is one of the aspect of the butterfly effect—chaos theory discussed in chapter 3).

People eat additional foods after having meals because they are hungry or their energy was stolen by environments around them (both internal and external). Armed with this knowledge, we should control the environments as we mentioned in chapter 4.

Additional foods such as cookies, bread, doughnuts, chocolate, or noodles are better taken four hours after your main meal (breakfast, lunch, and dinner), so you do not disturb the digestion process within that four-hour-period.

What if one day you have breakfast at 10:00 A.M., should you have your lunch at 12:00 P.M.? No, We know that digestion of a meal takes up to four hours, so it is better to have your lunch four or five hours after your breakfast, and your dinner, another four or five hours later. The next day you can have your breakfast at 7:00 A.M. as you normally do.

Balancing eating and sleeping

In previous chapter we mentioned the benefits of sleeping eight hours a day; these benefits include having a better digestive system because all the cells damaged during digestive process will be replaced by the new ones. Without enough sleep, those cells won't be recovered or renewed completely.

When we have sleep debt, we need to reduce foods especially those are difficult to digest such as meats (beef, pork, chicken), cheese, milk, junk foods, oily or fried foods. We should choose foods that can be digested easily such as vegetables, fruits, or fish. That's why many health books recommend eating more vegetables, fruits, and fish because people today find it difficult to sleep eight hours a day.

Sleeping is more important than eating, so it is better not to make an excuse to have sleep debt and compensate it with vegetables, fruits, and fish because we can have an accident caused by sleep debt. Also we never know how many pesticides or hormones are used to grow those vegetables or fruits and how many pollutants are in our fish.

If we sleep eight hours a day, our body will have enough energy to digest foods well, including beef, pork, and chicken, and we will seldom have any problems with our daily meals. So we should not assume that people who eat meats, cheese, or junk foods are not healthy or will die sooner than we will because we need to know how they sleep and also how often they eat those foods.

Several points to note:

- To find a suitable healthy food, you need to consult with a doctor or nutrition expert in your city or country because they will know your environment, health, activities, and foods available better than the health book authors. Health books are written by authors according to their environment, and their observations and the foods available in their environment may not be applicable to you.

- If a health book mentioned that certain foods are good for your health but those foods aren't grown in your country, you need to know why the food is still fresh after days or weeks of the delivery process. Are any preservatives used or will the vitamins or minerals be the same as ? Is that food within your budget; could a local food be substituted?

- There is no food for longevity in this world; each country has its own food composition.

- Actually, food is not more important than the other top three that make us healthy: air, sleep, and warm drinking water. God created us with the same air (oxygen) for breathing, night for sleeping, saliva or warm drinking water for quenching thirst, and different kind of foods in each country for eating; so when you are sick or have a disease such abnormal cells, diabetes, liver disease, or kidney disease, you should not blame your food only (unless it is poisonous). The top three with higher rank in command should be more responsible for your body. You should ask yourself "Do I have a clean air environment? Do I sleep eight hours a day? Do I drink warm water?"

- As food is not more important than those top three factors, you can pick any food compositions as recommended by various healthy food books or WHO recommendations, as long as it suits your health, environment, and activities.

Chapter 8

Our Body Guideline

When driving a car, we have a basic guideline on the road—the road line; we usually drive in between the road line and try not to cross that line and go off on the shoulder. Our body also needs guidelines, so we will know whether we are underweight, normal, overweight, or obese.

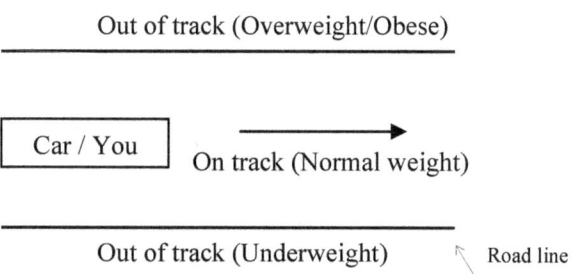

There is a simple and easy guideline called body mass index (BMI); it is a number calculated using a person's weight and height. BMI is an indicator of body fat, and we can consider it as an alternative to direct measures of body fat. BMI can give a rough indication whether we are on track or out of track because of the food we eat and our activity level. We may be eating too much or too little, not getting enough sleep, and leading a sedentary life.

BMI FORMULA

$$BMI = \frac{Weight\ (in\ Kg)}{Height \times Height\ (in\ Meter)}$$

BMI Measurement standard (for adult twenty-years-old or above) [4]

BMI Standard	Weight Status
Below 18.5	Underweight
18.5 – 24.9	Normal
25-29.9	Overweight
30 and above	Obese

For example:

If your body weight is 85 kg and your height is 1.8 Meter, your BMI is :

85 / (1.8 x 1.8) = 26.23 - OVERWEIGHT

---

[4] This standard isn't applicable to pregnant women, athletes, or children.

For this example, we cannot do much with the height; the only possible alteration is to change our weight by reducing it to normal level.

UNDERWEIGHT

Underweight is caused by spending more energy than you consume. There are several ways to solve this problem:

- Reducing activity level,
- Drink warm water when available
- Set the room temperature as close as 26° Celsius or 78.8° Fahrenheit,
- Sleep eight hours a day.

Adding food portions should be the last choice after reviewing and following the suggestions given above for one to three months. If you are underweight because of a disease, a doctor's advice is recommended to handle the disease first.

OVERWEIGHT AND OBESITY

Overweight and obesity are caused by expending less energy than you take in, which means you eat more than your body needs. It is true that you are have extra energy stored in your body in form of fat; but too much fat is not good, it adversely affect your heart, liver, and blood vessels (which are blocked by fat).

Overweight and Obese Circle

Based on my observations, there is an endless overweight or obese circle that may be applied to you.

Overweight or obese people usually need cold drinking water and cold room temperature because they have more energy to release (more fat); the more energy they release, the more food they want to eat. Eating more food will cause their digestive organs to work harder, which makes them sleepy, and this maintains or increases their weight.

Sometimes you may also notice that overweight or obese people tend to eat something near their bedtime; that's because they will be hungry if they do not eat any food. They will be hungry because the cold AC temperature takes a lot of their energy while they are sleeping.

Overweight or obese people tend to have more risk of body metabolism problems such as heart disease, liver disease, kidney disease, or digestive problems because they tend to drink cold water and eat more than other people; their digestive organs work harder than other people's.

If we look at the overweight and obese circle, we noticed that overweight and obese people tend to have cold drinking water and cold room temperature to accommodate the heat from their body, and as we know that cold temperature is one of external temperature that takes our energy and makes us hungry before eating time, we can modify the overweight and obese circle to overweight and obese *solution* circle.

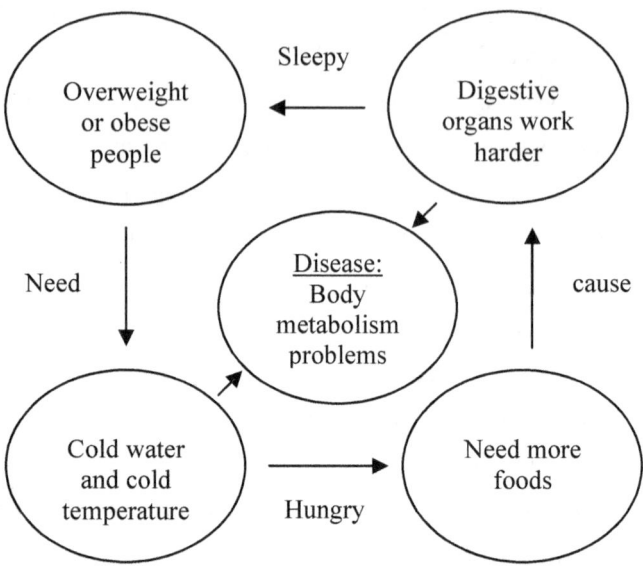

(Overweight and obese circle)

Overweight and Obese Solution Circle

In this overweight and obese solution circle, people need to drink warm water (36° to 37° Celsius or 96.8° to 98.6° Fahrenheit) and warm their room temperature incrementally to 26° Celsius (78.8° Fahrenheit). They will release less energy by having warm drinking water and adjusting their room temperature as close to 26° Celsius (78.8° Fahrenheit) as possible. If they release less energy, they will not feel too hungry at meal time (breakfast, lunch, dinner), and then they can reduce their meals by one-quarter to one-half of their current meal portions. Besides the reduction of meal portions, digestive organs can work better if they do not take any foods four hours after finishing their meal.

If the BMI measurement still shows that they're overweight after three months following this plan, portion size should be reduced by one-quarter to one-half. The meal reduction will make their digestive organs work better because there will be less food to digest. A better digestive system plus sweat baths will make them healthier (sweat baths can be replaced by regular exercise if the exercise makes them sweat).

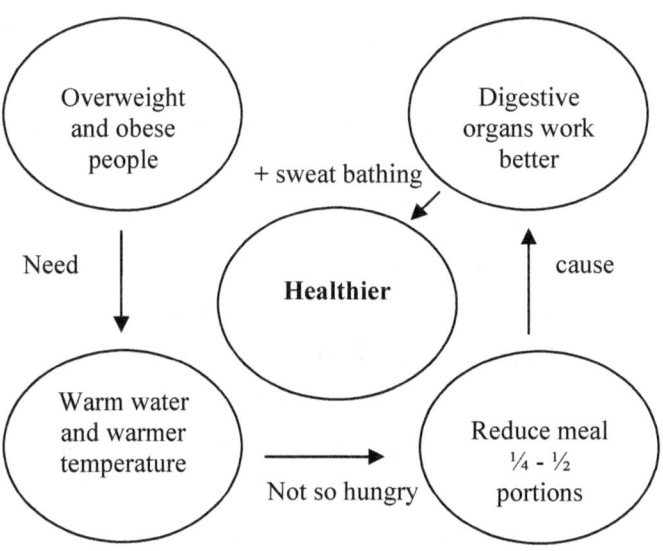

(Overweight and obese solution circle)

Chapter 9

SECRETS OF HEALTH = SECRETS OF WEALTH

Rich, John, Jim, and Betty are good friends; Rich is the richest among them. John, Jim, and Betty want to know how Rich is wealthy, so they try to find out his secrets the next time they visit his house.

Rich : *Hi, friends! What a surprise! What brings you here? Come in and have a seat.*

John : *Thanks, Rich, to be honest, we want to learn something from you. We want to know your wealthy secrets, so we can follow your way and become wealthy too. As our best friend, could you please let us know your secrets?*

Rich : *I do not have any wealthy secrets. I started my shop near my house and followed my father's advice; hmm... maybe my father's advice made me wealthy? Okay, I'll share it with you, but please you tell me what are you doing now?*

John : *I am a director of a big company*

Jim : *I am a manager of a medium-sized company*

Betty : *I am a secretary of a small company*

John : *All of us are working hard to become wealthy people, but we are still having the same financial problems, such as credit card debt and nothing left for savings. In other words, we would be almost bankrupt without financial aid from a bank loan.*

Rich : *Well, it is good news that all of you still have jobs and an income; John, you are a director, so your income must be higher than Jim's or Betty's. How could you have the same financial problems? Please, think again, what is your problem?*

John : *(Thirty minutes later) You are right Rich, my salary is higher than Jim's or Betty's, but I use my money to buy a new car every year, which I do for my image as a director of a big company.*

Jim : *I use my money for parties with my family after receiving my salary.*

Betty : *I use my money for buying expensive dresses after receiving my salary.*

Rich : *Hmm...now I am sure that my father's advice made me wealthy. Before I opened my shop, my father gave me several advice:*

- **When you receive money, save at least 10 percent**
- **Invest your money wisely**
- **Control your expenditures**
- **Make donation**

John : *Is that all?*

Rich : *Yes, that's all. Your financial problems are not caused by your income level but by expenditures. All of you have a source of income (money), but you do not invest or control it wisely. Instead, you spend your money for unnecessary things that do not grow your money. John is spending his money on cars that need maintenance. Jim is spending on monthly parties, and Betty is buying expensive dresses. You should spend your money on useful investments such as property, mutual funds, or gold, which can increase your wealth!*

Betty : *You are right, Rich; now we realize that we did not use our money wisely or control our expenditures. In the current financial crisis, my boss cannot do business anymore, and I won't be in the office next week.*

Jim : *Were you fired Betty?*

Betty : *Yes, now I am like a sick person—I am bankrupt! I cannot do anything other than thinking of my bad financial condition and credit card bills. I need another bank loan.*

Rich : *Don't worry, Betty. Now you know the wealthy secrets, when you get a job again, you can follow my father's advice. You can be wealthy too.*

That conversation emphasizes that having an income (money) is good and important, but it doesn't guarantee that you will be a wealthy person in the future. You must control your expenditures and invest your money wisely. John is a director, Jim is a manager, and Betty is a secretary; each has a different level of income but all are broke.

You may hear that a person who wins ten million dollars in a lottery is bankrupt the following year and wonder how that could possibly happen. It happened because the person did not use the money wisely or control his expenditures. It is not only the level of your income that makes you wealthy in the future but also how wisely you invest your money and control your expenditures.

The owner of a small restaurant can be wealthy if he invests his money and controls his expenditures to grow his wealth by buying other restaurants. A writer can be wealthy if he invests his money and controls his expenditures wisely to grow his wealth by buying and reading books to increase his skill and knowledge. A shoemaker can be wealthy if he invests his money, controls his expenditures wisely, and grows his wealth by opening a shoe factory. A poor farmer can be wealthy if he invests his money wisely, controls his expenditures, and grows his wealth by buying chickens and selling their eggs, and then using the proceeds to set up a chicken farm.

Everyone with any level of income can be wealthy if he or she invests wisely and controls expenditures. For a more extreme example, a thief can be wealthy if he invests his stolen money and controls his expenditures wisely to increase his wealth. Although there are more risks attached to this profession, and I do not recommend it.

Let's change that *wealthy secrets* conversation into a *healthy secrets* conversation:

Rich, John, Jim, and Betty are good friends; Rich is the healthiest among them. One day John, Jim and Betty are going to Rich's house to find out what the Rich's healthy secrets are.

Rich : *Hi, friends, what a surprise! What brings you here? Come in and have a seat.*

John : *Thanks, Rich. We want to learn your healthy secrets, so we can follow them and become healthy too. As our best friend, could you let us know your secrets?*

Rich : *I do not have any healthy secrets. I eat as usual, three times daily, and follow my father's advice; hmm...maybe my father's advice makes me healthy. Okay, I'll share with you, but can you tell me what you do for your health?*

John : *I follow a diet of healthy foods, exercise regularly, and avoid junk food.*

Jim : *I am a vegetarian and exercise twice a month.*

Betty : *I eat any food, take vitamins, and exercise once in a while.*

John : *All of us are trying hard to keep healthy, but we still get sick and some times cannot go to work. In other words, all of us could die if we didn't take medicines prescribed by a doctor.*

Rich : *Well, it is good news that all of you are still eating. John, you eat a healthy diet and exercise regularly,* surely you must be healthier than Jim and Betty? How could you get sick too? Please consider what might be your problem.

John : *(Thirty minutes later) You are right, Rich, I exercise regularly and eat right, but I usually don't get to sleep until 1:00 A.M. and wake up at 6:00 A.M. for my job.*

Jim : *I like to drink cold water and beer; once in a while, I get drunk.*

Betty : *My husband is fat, and he usually sets our bedroom temperature at 17° Celsius (62.6° Fahrenheit), otherwise he can't sleep.*

Rich : *Hmm....now I am sure that my father's advice makes me healthy. When I was young, my father gave me several bits of advice:*

- **Have enough sleep (eight hours) and drink warm water to save your energy**
- **Use/invest your energy wisely**
- **Control your released energy**
- **Spend some energy for social life/activity**

John : *Is that all?*

Rich : *Yes, that's all. Your health problems are not caused by your eating habits, they are dependent on how wisely you use and control your energy. All of you have enough energy, but you do not use and control it wisely; instead, you use and release your energy for unnecessary things that do not have a positive impact on your health. John is using his energy for staying up*

79

late and only sleeps five hours to recover his energy.
Jim's energy is used for absorbing the cold water and
alcohol in his body, and Betty's energy is used for
adapting to the cold temperature in her bedroom. You
should use your energy for something that can increase
your health such as walking in the morning, practicing
Tai Chi, practicing normal sweat bathing, reading
health books, laughing and smiling (be happy), etc.

Betty : *You are right Rich. Now we realized that we do not use*
wisely and control our energy. I also have bad temper
with my husband because he doesn't want to
understand me, and now my doctor said that I may have
cancer.

Jim : *Is it serious Betty?*

Betty : *It is only an indication of cancer, however I am a sick*
person now, and I cannot do anything other than think
of my disease. I need to take a lot of medicines.

Rich : *Don't worry, Betty. Now you know the healthy secrets,*
so you can keep eating your foods for energy and follow
my father's advice. You can be healthy too.

From that conversation, we can learn that eating healthy foods is important, but to be healthy in the future, there are other more important factors—use your energy wisely and control your released energy.

John, Jim, and Betty are eating healthy foods, but they are in poor health because they do not use and control their energy wisely to increase their health. There was a young actor who was in good health and then fell sick and died recently because he was so influenced by a character in a film that he experienced stress, insomnia, and then took sleeping pills. This happened because he did not use and control his energy wisely; **it is not only the foods you eat that make you healthy in the future but how wisely you use and control your energy.**

Vegetarian menus, food-combining menus, food based on blood type menus, or current daily menus can also make people healthy in the future if they always use and control the released energy to increase their health. This includes sleeping for eight hours, drinking warm water, having regular exercise, controlling negative emotions, etc. A junk food menu can also make people healthy in the future if they use and control their energy wisely. Although there are more risks associated with eating this food, but there is no guarantee that these individuals will die or get sick faster than people who eat healthy foods. (I do not recommend this extreme diet.)

Secrets of Wealth	Secrets of Health
From the money you earned, save at least 10 percent	**From the food you eat, which generate your energy:**
• If you save 10 percent from your income, you are richer than those who never save money.	• Sleep for eight hours a day to save your energy; you will have more energy than those who do not sleep eight hours

	Drink warm water to save energy; you will have more energy than those who never drink warm water.
Invest your money wisely • Invest your money to increase your wealth, i.e. property, mutual fund, gold, time deposits, etc.	**Use/invest your energy wisely** • Use your energy to increase your health, i.e. regular walking thirty minutes a day, practicing Tai Chi, laughing, reading health books, etc.
Control your expenditure • Make sure that you are aware that a luxurious lifestyle can take your money. You should control your lifestyle, so you can control your money.	**Control your released energy** • Make sure that you are aware of external and internal environments than can take your energy. You should control your environments so you can control your released energy.
Make donations • It is mentioned by God "*man shall not live by bread alone, but by every word of God,*" and every word of God is "**LOVE.**" Life is not just about money; you need to share with others and show your love by helping them. It	**Spend some energy for social life or activity** • It is mentioned by God "*man shall not live by bread alone, but by every word of God,*" and every word of God is "**LOVE.**" You cannot express your love by living alone in your apartment or house. You need

is more blessed to give than to receive. You will receive more wealth by giving than receiving.	to be with other people talking, smiling, laughing, and sharing. If you give one smile to 10 people, you will get 10 smiles back.

Explanations:

- **Having enough sleep (eight hours in a day) and drinking warm water to save your energy**

  In chapter 6 we discussed the mathematic calculation for sleep debt—simplified. Energy wasted if we do not sleep eight hours a day; in other words, we can save the wasted energy in our body if we get eight hours of sleep. We will have more energy than other people who do not sleep eight hours a day.

  In chapter 3, we calculated the effect of the energy lost by drinking cold water; here we can say that you still have more energy than other people who do not drink warm water. The lost energy from drinking cold water is actually not only in our stomach; there are other organs such as the pancreas, liver, and small intestines that are also affected by cold temperature, and this is caused by the conduction of liquid material factor. If you are still in doubt about the value of lost energy from drinking cold water, you can ask your doctor's advice about drinking cold water when you are sick or have a fever.

- **Use/invest your energy wisely**

  Spending energy is fun because it is similar to spending money; we need to spend energy in our daily life, but it is wiser to spend it in activities that can increase our health such as walking around thirty minutes a day, practicing Tai Chi, reading health books, laughing, smiling, cleaning unhealthy room environments, etc.

  Spending energy for smoking, drinking alcohol, taking drugs, chatting, browsing the Internet, or other activities that reduce our sleeping time are examples of using energy unwisely.

  A person who has been bankrupt tends to have more appreciation of his money when he recovers his wealth. This is similar to the heightened appreciation of his energy someone who was gravely ill has when he recovers his health. So it is better to spend and invest our energy wisely before it is too late to appreciate it.

- **Control your released energy**

  There are external environments such as room temperature, outside weather, and internal environments such as negative emotions (chapter 3 and 4) that can steal our energy, make us hungry before meal time, and push us to eat more. If we can control the energy released because of the environments, we can reduce our meals and help our digestive organs work better.

- **Spend some energy for social life or activity**

  People need love from others and to give love to others. To receive and give love, we can't be in our apartment or house alone. We need families or friends to talk, share, and laugh. When we are young, social life usually is not an issue because we are still working and have friends. The situation may be different when we are old, retired, and our children are have their own families; we could be end up in alone spending most of our time watching TV and browsing the Internet. This situation is not healthy and can make us stressed, depressed and insomniacs; all the diseases start from there.

  Having a social life or sharing activities with friends or meeting people when we are old can help us avoid some negative emotions. A good social life also makes us sleep well. Some social life or activities can be:
  - open a small business so we can talk, share, and laugh with friends or clients,
  - join a religious organization or charity organization so we can smile and share love with others,
  - any other activities that can keep us meeting and communicating with other people.

Chapter 10

Chance to Live More Than 100 Years

For centuries, people have sought foods that would ensure longevity. Ginseng, bird nest, yogurt, milk, enzymes, vitamins, and green tea are frequently mentioned as good for longevity, but they do not solve the longevity issue.

Most people want to know the secrets of the person who can reach 100-years-old or more; people want to know what that person eats and drinks. If he/she drinks milk, people will conclude that drinking milk can prolong life; if he/she is a vegetarian or ingests yogurt, green tea, or ginseng, people will conclude that being a vegetarian or ingesting yogurt, green tea, or ginseng guarantees a long life.

Actually, there are other factors that can take human life such as accidents, diseases caused by viruses or bacteria, and diseases caused by body metabolism problems; these factors are the issues we need to solve before talking about longevity.

For poor and developing countries, most of their health issues are caused by viruses or bacteria; for wealthy countries, their health issues are mostly caused by body metabolism problems such as high cholesterol, abnormal cells, heart attack, diabetes, liver disease, kidney disease, etc.

Many health book authors have explained how those health issues can happen; they also propose several foods to eat or avoid and a set the percentage of each food group that should be consumed, e.g., 68 percent carbohydrates, 10 percent protein, and 22 percent fat. Each author has his own argument and observations, no one is 100 percent wrong. We must appreciate their information about healthy foods.

From those food compositions, you can choose one that suits your eating style. Why can't you choose the best food composition? Each is touted as the best, so how can you choose? No books can give you the best food formula because your living environment, activities, and health conditions may be different from those of the authors. You need to pay attention to whether the books mentioned that you should not eat meat or junk food or cheese or other foods for many reasons. You can improve your health by reducing the amount of those foods that you eat.

We can't be perfect by eating the right the foods because foods are not the only factor in our health system; there are other factors and habits that make us healthy and increase our chance to live to be more than 100-years-old.

The chart below gives more information on how the health system works in our life and how to increase you chance of living to be 100-years-old.

Chance to live more than 100 years chart:

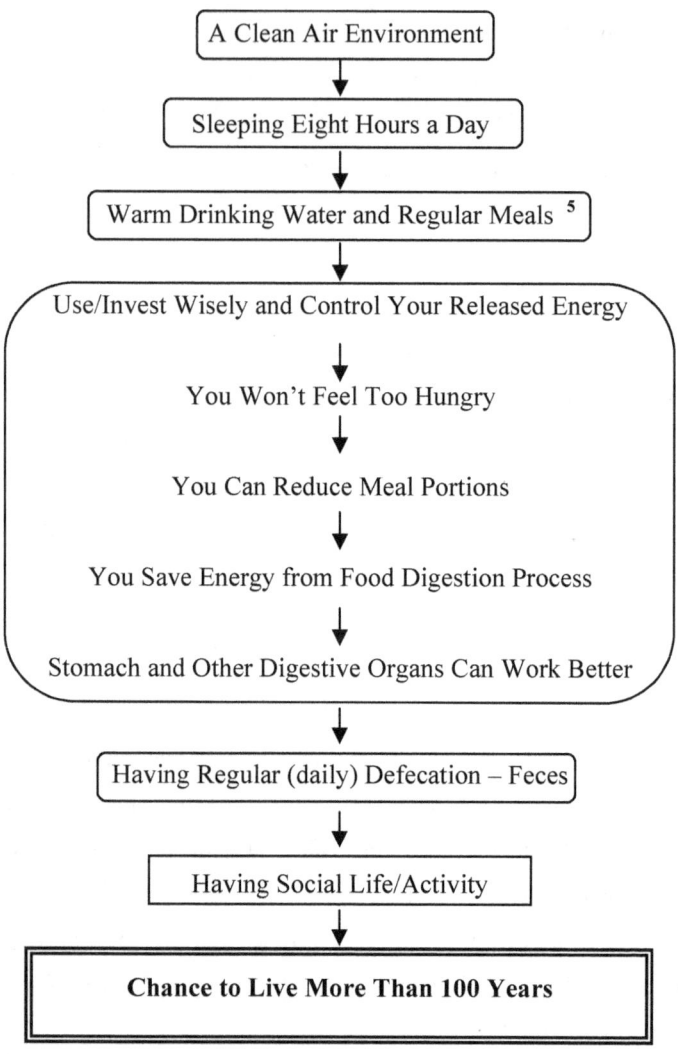

A Clean Air Environment

↓

Sleeping Eight Hours a Day

↓

Warm Drinking Water and Regular Meals [5]

↓

Use/Invest Wisely and Control Your Released Energy

↓

You Won't Feel Too Hungry

↓

You Can Reduce Meal Portions

↓

You Save Energy from Food Digestion Process

↓

Stomach and Other Digestive Organs Can Work Better

↓

Having Regular (daily) Defecation – Feces

↓

Having Social Life/Activity

↓

Chance to Live More Than 100 Years

---

[5] Healthy foods are recommended for your meals. If you don't know what are healthy foods, you can eat your current foods for meals (do not change your meals).

Explanations:

- Air (oxygen) is very important in our life; we can die if we do not breathe for a few minutes. Air is used to generate energy in our body and clean air can give better energy for our body.

- Sleeping eight hours a day is recommended. You can read again chapter 6 about The Secret of Sleeping for its benefits. Sleeping is the process of energy distribution to all your body and this process is controlled by your brain; your brain needs rest to better control the systems in your body. No matter how healthy your food is, if you don't sleep well, you can get sick easily.

- Having a meal and drinking warm water are good for your body energy, and it is recommended that you eat healthy foods for your meals; if you are not sure about which are healthy foods; you can stick to your current meals menu and do not change it.

- Use/invest wisely and control your released energy to prevent you from wasting energy. There are external and internal environments that can waste your energy, and you need to control them (i.e., set room temperature as close as $26°$ Celsius or $78.8°$ Fahrenheit, reduce negative emotions, etc., see chapter 4). I would suggest you also invest your energy in reading more health books written by doctors or nutritionists to increase your health. You only need to pay attention to the foods they recommend you to avoid and then reduce the amount of those foods in your diet. You don't have to avoid all those foods because they may not be 100 percent right.

Once you know what you should avoid, then you can increase your skill by knowing what you should add to your meals. However, if you don't like the new foods, don't push yourself to eat them.

- Once you sleep eight hours a day and control your released energy, you won't feel too hungry at breakfast, lunch, or dinner.

- If you are not so hungry, you can reduce your meal portions by around one-quarter to one-half from your normal meals and try not to eat within four hours after your meals.

- When reducing meal portions, you automatically reduce the energy needed for digesting food such as physical process (chewing, stomach, and intestines digestve process) and chemical process (energy to produce enzymes in saliva, stomach, liver, and pancreas).

  Imagine that a person who usually lifts a 30 Kgs box is asked to lifs 20 Kgs box,. He can do it easily and spends less energy; imagine that your stomach usually digests 300 grams of food, and then you give it only 200 grams of food to digest. Your stomach can do it easily and spends less energy too.

- Reducing your meal portions also makes your stomach and other digestive organs work better because they digest less food; all the digestive enzymes can be mixed well into your food.

- Defecation [6] is the last process of the whole digestive process. This part plays an important role in your life, and you should

---

[6] Urine and other excretions are not included to simplify the explanation.

not miss this part of daily life. If you have a defecation problem (constipation), I would point to your sleeping habits first before your food as the main cause of this problem. (That is in the absence of certain disease or certain medicines that make one prone to constipation.) If you have meals three times a day, and it takes about thirty minutes for each meal, it shouldn't be an issue for you to spend thirty minutes for defecation a day. You can read a book/newspaper or listen to radio during this activity. I know that some of you may be screaming for these thirty minutes, but the point is not thirty minutes; that is just an illustration. The point is not to be in a hurry to complete this activity because of work or other demands of life.

- Social life/activity is not part of body functions; it is a kind of communication with other people. We need friends or family to talk or share or laugh. Opening a small business or joining an organization when we are old can keep us meeting and communicating with other people.

Why is reaching more than 100-years-old difficult?

1. Air Pollution

There is no compromise on air pollution because air (oxygen) is very important for your health. You cannot control the outside air environment, but you can control the air in your environments—bedroom, office room, meeting room, etc.

Smoke from cigarettes is one cause of air pollution, and you should have a solution with your partner if your bedroom is full of smoke because this will affect your health in the future. Your health is important to enjoy your life; if you are not wealthy today, it doesn't mean you cannot be very wealthy in the future because now you know how to transmit your wishes clearly for your wealth and health (chapter 6).

2. **People do not sleep eight hours a day**

The modern lifestyle, with its dreams, workload, and stress, makes it hard to get eight hours of sleep a day; without adequate sleep, the brain does not have enough time to replace old cells with the new cells. As the war general of your body, the brain also needs rest to control the distribution and absorption of energy from food. Without enough energy, your body can't handle the viruses, bacteria, abnormal cells, side effects of medicines, or neutralize any pesticides or pollutants in your body.

3. **People do not drink warm water**

As explained in a previous chapter, cold drinking water or ice water will change the digestive enzymes and chyme temperature in our stomach. As liquids, chyme and enzymes are good conductors, especially when they are mixed with water. (Imagine a cup of hot coffee to which you add cold water; the coffee's temperature will be affected.) They can transfer the cold temperature to other parts of digestive organs such as intestines, liver, pancreas, etc., and this inhibits the work of the enzymes and hormones in those organs. People of all ages should drink warm water regardless of the external or internal temperature.

4. People eat too much at a meal

People overeat because they are hungry or they need more energy to do their activities well.

In daily life, some energy is actually wasted because of the environments (external and internal), and that's why they need more food to replace the wasted energy; eating more food means extra work for the stomach and other digestive organs. If people can control the environments (external and internal), they do not have to eat as much at a meal, and this will be good for the stomach and other digestive organs. Reducing the amount you eat can also reduce the pesticides, preservatives, or other chemical materials in vegetables, fruits, rice, fishes, meats, sugar, etc. in your body.

The older you are, the less food you should eat because your metabolic process is slower. (Some estimate this process starts to slow at age thirty.) This means that if you are fifty-years-old, you should not eat as much as someone twenty-five-years-old.

5. People do not have a social life/activity when they are old

Doing things with friends or family such as opening a small business, exercising together (walking in the morning), or engaging in positive activities (things that can make us smile, share our love, and sleep well) can be beneficial when we are old. Spending time with other people helps one feel both needed and not alone in this world.

Being lonely can cause people to feel stressed and may lead to depression. All these emotions are negative and take a lot of energy. The health problems usually start when those negative emotions cause sleeping problems.

Once we know how important feeling connected is, we can start visiting or telephoning our parents and grandparents once a week. You can ask about their activities or health conditions. Our visit or phone call lets them know that we care about and love them, so they can sleep well. It is better to spend a few dollars on phone calls than thousands of dollars for their medical treatment! (*just joking*)

From all those explanations, we can say that you are:
- Where you breathe
- How you sleep
- What you drink and eat
- When you defecate (feces)
- Who your friends and family are

Chapter 11

The Next Wars

Lucy and Anne are having discussion on the terrorist attack.

Lucy   : Are we at war now?

Anne   : Yes, we are.

Lucy   : But our country seems quiet and peaceful.

Anne   : Did you visit a hospital in the last thirty days?

Lucy   : No, what happened?

Anne   : Hospitals are more crowded than hotels!

Lucy   : What happened?

Anne   : We are at war now.

Lucy   : ???#@!

When we mention war, people usually think about war against terrorism, conventional war, or nuclear war; actually in daily life, we have bigger wars than those wars. Most people are more interested in terrorist attacks that killed 200 people in a year than heart attacks that kill 2,000 people in a day!

The wars inside the human body are bigger and last longer than World War I or II; the funny thing is people do not realize that they have wars in their body.

There are two kinds of wars in our body:

1. War against viruses and bacteria

Each year, new viruses or bacteria are discovered from human body, and many diseases are attributed to them. The research on viruses and bacteria is an endless task because there are millions of them that still haven't been named. Also, they can mutate anytime, and the mutation can occur more quickly with the side effects of medicines. We cannot control the new creation of those viruses or bacteria in this world, but we still can keep our energy steady, so our body's immune system will be at the highest level all the time.

The war against viruses and bacteria will be harder in future because of global warming. Global warming may change the climate or weather in this world, and it won't be a surprise if in the next couple of years, new deadly viruses or bacteria are discovered. The changes of climate or weather will take our energy to adapt with the environment, and that will have impact to our body's immune system.

The strength of future viruses or bacteria may be the same as current strength; it is the changes of climate or weather that make us lose more energy (if we do not control it) and lack energy to support the immune system. People will assume that viruses or bacteria are stronger, but indeed our body is weaker because we waste more energy on the environments and start eating more.

2. War against body metabolism problems

For rich countries or rich people, the war against body metabolism problems is a bigger war than the war against viruses or bacteria; most of these people face kidney disease, heart disease, liver disease, lung disease, digestive problems, etc. that are caused by their eating and sleeping habits.

This war is a little bit silent because you won't know your afflicted until you have tests of your blood, urine, feces, and other medical tests. This month you may have a good result, but in the next few months, you may have a different result. Some people do not like to visit a doctor and usually wait until they are having problems with their health. Having regular medical screening is the first step to prevent bigger health problems in future.

The next wars

The biggest issue for the next war is that people will be battling wars against viruses or bacteria and metabolic problems at the same time; these will be the next deadly wars.

If we have two kinds of wars in our body at the same time, the chance to win the wars are small; and you probably lose the war or die. A bigger chance to win the wars is to have only one war or make the other war as small as possible.

We cannot stop the war against viruses and bacteria because they are around us every day, but we can stop or make the war against metabolic problems as small as possible. So, it is important for you to choose the war-winning strategies.

How to win the war against viruses or bacteria?

Strategy: **The Healthy Secrets (chapter 9):**

- Have enough sleep (eight hours a day) and drink warm water to save your energy
- Use your energy wisely
- Control the released energy
- Spend some energy for social life/activity

How to win or minimize the war against metabolic problems?

Strategy: **Chance to live more than 100 Years (chapter 10)**

- A clean air environment
- Sleep for eight hours a day
- Do not eat too much (reduce your meals)
- Regular defecation (feces)

Although we have shared the healthy secrets and chance to live more than 100 years, there is no guarantee you will win the wars against viruses or bacteria and metabolic problems. Those two wars' strategies are intended to give you enough body energy for a steady immune system that's working at the highest level. You will have a better preparation from "enemy" attacks than those who do not have any strategies for the wars; this means that if you are sick, you can recover faster, i.e., in three days when others will need three weeks or even three months.

Do you need equipment for the next wars?

It is better you prepare equipment for the next wars; the equipment is **Fruit**. You can have your local fruits such as an orange, apple, strawberry, pear, mango, grape, kiwi, or banana, depending on your health conditions. However, I would suggest you do not forget one fruit—**Papaya** (or other similar food if papayas are not available in your city).

Why Papaya fruit?

Papaya fruit has natural vitamins and enzymes that are good for your digestive system—especially vitamin C and the papain enzyme. If you want to learn more about this fruit, you can search the Internet with Google or Yahoo using the keywords *papaya benefit*. You will be surprised to learn that papaya fruit, with its vitamins and enzymes, is also good for your heart, blood vessels, lungs, immune system, bones, etc.

You can have this fruit several times a week with other fruits, and it is better you eat fresh fruits not dried or canned fruits.

The reasons we need to eat papaya fruit:

a. It can treat digestive disorders and constipation problems. Recent research revealed that healthy digestive system is one of the keys to a healthy life.

b. This fruit can grow easily without the use of many pesticides or growth hormones.

c. The fruit can be imported without using any chemical protection; it can be imported raw.

Another fruit that you should consider is **pineapple.**

Pineapple is good for the digestive system, and Chinese people believe that this fruit is a natural colon cleaner. This fruit, which contains natural antioxidants and vitamin C, is also good for bones, constipation, and blood clotting problems. For those who have chronic stomach problems, please be careful with this fruit because it may trigger a heavy stomachache; your doctor's advice is recommended before eating this fruit. Pineapple fruit is better served after your meals, and a few slices of this fruit should be enough in a week.

There is a pro and contra on the negative effects of papaya and pineapple fruits for pregnant women or women who plan to have a baby. In these cases, it is better to avoid these fruits or seek a doctor's advice before eating these fruits.

When is the best time to eat fruit?

Some health books recommend that you eat fruit before a meal and the others recommend that you eat fruit after a meal. I would prefer having fruit after a meal, and there are several reasons for this:

1. Your fruit may be fresh from refrigerator. When you eat it before meal, it is still cold and this may cause temperature

shock to your stomach. If you eat fruit after a meal, your meal can absorb some of the fruit's temperature in the stomach. Alternatively, you can chew the cold fruit a bit longer in your mouth to make it a little bit warmer.

2. Your fruit may taste sweet in your mouth, but after several enzymes processes in your mouth and stomach, it can become sour or uncomfortable for your stomach; some of these fruits are pineapple, mango, orange, kiwi, strawberry. By having these fruits after meal, you reduce risk of stomach irritation by those fruits.

Eat fresh fruit or drink fresh fruit juice?

If time permitted, it is better to eat fresh fruit because we still have time to chew the fruit to make it a bit warm for our stomach and also to let the enzymes in our mouth work. Drinking fresh fruit juice is similar to eating fresh fruit, however if we still have a choice, it is better not to drink it at cold temperature (or with ice); adding some hot water (a few spoonfuls) to make it a little bit warm is a good idea. Drinking cold fruit juice is actually worse than drinking plain cold water because fruit juice particles can remain cold longer than plain water.

Do you need a coalition to win the wars?

If you think that you will lose the wars or have heavy destruction, it is better to have coalitions from one or several parties such as doctors, nutrition experts, psychologists, etc. Of course, the coalition is not free, but it is better than losing the war or having heavy destruction in your body. Don't be negative or stubborn about having a coalition, otherwise you will be captured by the enemies and stay in their prison without hope of release.

There are also other issues in human health that are out of our control such as accidents, nuclear/radioactive radiations, and congenital abnormalities; for these issues we really need coalitions.

Are you ready for the next wars?

In the future or now, the wars are triggered by you and not by the enemies. You declare war while you are unprepared for the wars!

Twenty–four-hour lifestyles that make you unconsciously declare the wars include:

- Twenty-four-hour Internet availability and social networking Web sites
- Twenty-four-hour online games
- Twenty-four-hour TV channels
- Twenty-four-hour financial market, i.e., foreign exchange market.
- Twenty-four-hour mobile phones on standby in our bedroom
- Twenty-four-hour restaurants and delivery service
- Other twenty-four-hour services

These kinds of services will take most of your sleeping time, make you hungry, and cause you to eat more food. Eating more food, especially before bedtime, will make your digestive organs work harder when they should take a rest. This situation will affect your digestive system and cause metabolic problems in the long term.

There is nothing wrong with all those services (actually they are very helpful), but we need to know our energy limitation for enjoying those things. We can calculate easily the hours of sleeping after having those services and see whether we have much sleep debt and try to pay it as soon as possible..

By knowing all these things, we should be careful with daily habits in the future because besides the twenty-four-hour services, the climate changes (global warming) will take additional energy from our body and make us unprepared for the wars.

Knowledge on Healthy life is as important as Wealthy life

Most parents teach their children about money by buying financial books for them and giving advice such as save your money, spend your money wisely, have some investments, etc. However, financial knowledge is not enough for children's future, we need to teach them about the concept of energy and digestive system in the human body, so they know how to save their energy, use/invest their energy wisely, and control the released energy. This knowledge will put their body at the highest protection level from viruses or bacteria or metabolic problems in the future. We need to teach them early because health is built with daily habits.

A wealthy family does not guarantee a transfer of healthy-life knowledge to their children. We can notice that some wealthy families do not pay serious attention to their children's health and let them continue in obese or overweight conditions, take cold water, have cold room temperature, have alcohol or drugs, smoke, or have twenty-four-hour services in their bedroom. Often, parents don't discuss with their children the negative effects of twenty-four-hour services on the body. If they are not aware, all these things will have negative impacts on the children's future because they unconsciously declare the wars without any preparation. It is our duty as parents to let them know the secrets of health in addition to the secrets of wealth.

Chapter 12

Ideas on Healthy Equipment

We have gone through several steps in this book such as sweat bathing, drink warm water, and have a clean air environment, however in daily life, sometimes there is no room in a hospital for sweat bathing, there is no warm water available in our room, and it is difficult to know the air quality in our environment. With those difficulties, there are several ideas on new healthy equipment that should be available for practical and healthy reasons.

1. Adult incubator

A weak or premature baby is usually placed in an incubator and there are several reasons for that:

- Incubator can keep the temperature the same as mother's womb temperature
- Incubator can support a premature baby's undeveloped nervous system and help them grow faster.

An adult incubator (without ultraviolet lamp or UV) is similar to a baby incubator; we just change the size to fit adults. This equipment makes sweat bathing for adult people who are sick at home or hospital easy. Using an adult incubator for a patient should be under a doctor's recommendation and should be based on the patient's health condition.

The benefits of adult incubator are (same as sweat bathing):
- It will take out toxins from our body.
- It will make our body hot but exceed body temperature, and this will increase our blood circulation.
- It will reduce our kidneys' job of cleaning blood

2. Drinking water dispenser with *healthy* option

Our definition for healthy drinking water is drinking water at 36° to 37° Celsius (96.8° to 98.6° Fahrenheit).

In normal water dispensers, there are only hot and cold options. We need to add *healthy* option to those drinking water dispensers, so people or patients can get the standard warm water easily. The *healthy* option will give drinking water at 36° to 37° Celsius (96.8° to 98.6° Fahrenheit) temperature.

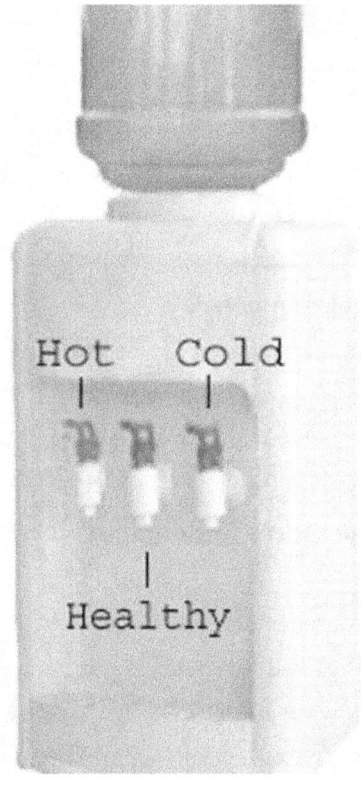

(A water dispenser with *healthy* option with temperature
36°to 37° Celsius or 96.8° to 98.6° Fahrenheit)

3. Glass with thermometer or indicator that shows healthy temperature level

Other alternatives for people who do not want to change their current water dispenser is a glass with thermometer or lamp / LED or other indicator that can give healthy or warm temperature indicator. We need this kind of indicator because sometimes we can have water that is too hot or too cold when we mix it manually from a normal water dispenser.

4. Spoon with thermometer

A spoon with a thermometer can be good equipment when we travel because we could measure our drinking water's temperature instantly.

5. Healthy temperature button or switch at water heater machines.

It takes several attempts for us to set the suitable water temperature when we are taking a bath at home, hotel, or hospital from a water heater machine; we need to use trial and error to find the correct water temperature. However, if there was a button or switch to set healthy or warm temperature at 36 to 37° Celsius (96.8° to 98.6° Fahrenheit) automatically, it will be very helpful.

6. Watch or Clock or Mobile Phone that can show room temperature

People usually look at their watch or clock or short message (SMS) but seldom look at their room temperature; external environment such as room temperature can waste our energy and make us hungry before meals. If the room temperature is hot, we can feel it and start complaining. But if the room temperature is cold, we seldom complain. By having a watch or clock or mobile phone that displays the room temperature clearly, we will know how strong the external temperature is, and then we can take some action to control that environment.

7. Portable air quality meter

With a portable air quality meter we can measure the air quality index or air pollution index in an environment before we rent or buy a house or an apartment. This equipment should be small like a compass or installed in a mobile phone.

A portable air quality meter will make property developers aware of the air quality in their project. If they are not aware, people with this equipment can make a decision not to invest in their properties. I believe this equipment can motivate people and corporations to create green environments by reducing or controlling pollution and planting more trees in their environment. This would help reduce the global warming process. Without a portable air quality meter, how can we know the air quality around us? How do we care about the global warming?

8. Mini or Pocket oxygen generator or purifier

A mini or pocket oxygen generator or purifier will be useful for sick people, especially when they are going out for some reason. This equipment would be even more useful if it were combined with a portable air quality meter (see no. 7), so we can use this equipment when the air quality is bad. People who work in environments with heavy air pollution such as policemen, miners, factory workers, and drivers will benefit from this equipment.

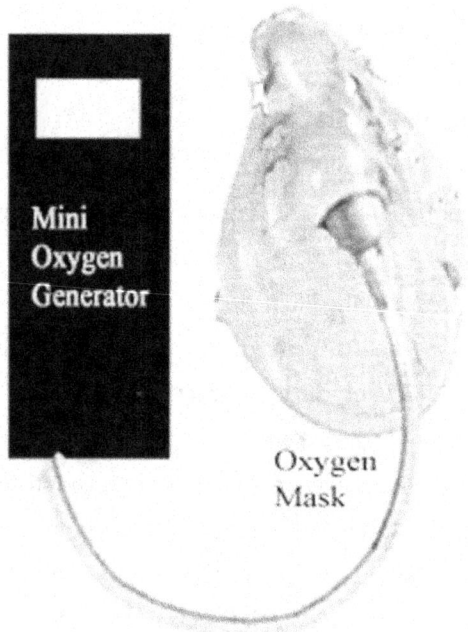

Mini Oxygen Generator & Mask

9. Sleep debt meter

If you have credit card debt, you can go to the bank and ask customer service for a list of your debt. What about your sleep debt? You should be able go to a hospital or a doctor to check your overall sleep debt with a sleep debt meter. This new equipment should give us our total sleep debt by checking various bodily functions, so we can take some action before it is too late to pay the debt. This equipment is quite useful for pilots, drivers, miners, and machine operators, so they can minimize some work accidents.

- 0 -

The Summary

- 0 -

Chapter 13

Summary

There are two kinds of wars in human health system:

a. War against viruses and bacteria

b. War against metabolic problems

To win the wars, you need two strategies that are secrets of health and chance to live to be more than 100-years-old. Although these strategies do not guarantee that you will win the wars, but at least you will have a better chance to win or minimize the impact from the wars; your body's immune system can function at the highest level to protect you from any diseases.

Secrets of health:

- Have enough sleep (eight hours a day) and drink warm water. to save your energy.
- Use/invest your energy wisely.
- Control the released energy.
- Spend some energy for social life/activity.

Chance to live more than 100 years:

- A clean air environment.
- Sleep for eight hours a day.
- Do not eat too much (reduce your meals).
- Regular defecation (feces).

There are several steps of exercises that can cover secrets of health and chance to live more than 100 years.

A. **Measure your BMI (Body Mass Index – see chapter 8)**

B. **Basic steps**
    1. Try to sleep for eight hours at night.
    2. Try to drink warm water when available.
    3. Try to eat fresh fruits every day.
    4. Try to defecate (feces) every day.

C. **Intermediate steps**
    1. Run basic step.
    2. Try to reduce your meals (breakfast, lunch, and dinner) by one-quarter to one-half.
    3. Try not to eat anything for four hours after your meal except fruits and warm water.
    4. Try to set room temperature as close to 26˚ Celsius (78.8˚ Fahrenheit)as possible, if not possible, try to adjust your clothes.

D. **Advance steps**

1. Run basic and intermediate steps.

2. Try to have a morning walk of at least thirty minutes regularly with your family or friends (better under morning sunlight); you can choose other exercises.

3. Try to invest your time wisely by reading more health books written by doctors or nutrition experts. Look for food you need to reduce and add or try to have a consultation with doctors or nutrition expert for advice about your healthy meals.

4. Try to have regular medical screening.

E. **Optional steps**

1. Try to invest in an air/oxygen purifier or AC with oxygen purifier (if this is available and within your budget).

2. Try to wear sandals or socks or shoes if the floor is cold or hot.

3. If you are still overweight after three months following those steps, you can try to reduce your meal portions by another one-quarter to one-half - please consider your health condition first.

4. Try to control your negative emotions.

5. Try to take warm water for bathing especially when you are tired or sick or bathing at night.

6. If you have a physical disability, try sweat bathing several times a month

7. Try to have a social life or engage in activities by building good relationships with other people.

Measuring BMI can give you an indicator of how you drive your body; it should be within normal range.

The basic step is to prepare yourself for war against viruses and bacteria (which is your daily war).

The intermediate step is to prepare yourself for war against metabolic problems.

The advance step is to prepare yourself to invest in something that can increase your health.

The optional step is something that you can consider if it is not an issue for you.

The Secret of Sleeping

The secret of secrets in human life is sleeping for eight hours a day. Let's start praying to God or the universe when we wake up in the morning after eight hours of sleep and wish for health and wealth in our life.

You are not only what you eat, but **you are:**
- Where you breathe
- How you sleep
- What you drink and eat
- When you defecate (feces)
- Who your friends and family are

Balancing eating and sleeping

Balancing eating and sleeping can lower the risk of metabolic problems. When you have sleep debt, try to eat foods that can be digested easily such as vegetables, fruits, and fish, and reduce the amount of meat (chicken, beef, and pork), milk, cheese, junk foods, oily or fried foods you eat.

Remember these:

- Having sleep debt and cold drinking water are the root of metabolic and immune system problems.
- Viruses or bacteria are smaller than an ant; you are bigger and stronger than an ant. Just blow the virus or bacteria out from your body, and it will go away.

Chapter 14

Jokes

In a classroom

Teacher : *Do you know what is the difference between healthy and wealthy?*

Tom : *Yes, sir, the difference is the H and W in front of those words.*

Teacher : *#@$, Which one is more important?*

Lucy : *Healthy, sir!*

Teacher : *Why, Lucy?*

Lucy : *Because H is in front of W in alphabet, sir!*

Teacher : *#@&*! Okay class, let's take a break now.*

In a senior high school classroom:

Teacher : *Can you mention some unhealthy foods, Bill?*

Bill : *Beans, vegetables, apple, rice, milk, and fish.*

Students : *Ha...ha....Stupid!! ...Idiot!!... Those are healthy foods!*

Teacher	:	*Can you mention some of healthy foods, Bill?*
Bill	:	*Beans, vegetables, apple, rice, milk, and fish.*
Teacher	:	*That is right, Bill, but why did you mention the same things for unhealthy foods?*
Bill	:	*Because both my father and my grandmother eat beans, vegetables, apple, rice, milk, and fish. But my father died at age fifty because of kidney disease, and my ninety-five-year-old grandmother has been healthy all her life. My grandmother cooks for us every day.*
Teacher	:	*I...I...think you are quite right for those two answers, Bill...... Hmm....*
Students	:	*What??*

A very rich man and his girlfriend are walking in a garden

Man	:	*I have made a decision to marry you. What about you?*
Girlfriend	:	*Hmm..I need more time to think about it.*
Man	:	*After spending five years together, you need more time to think about our relationship???*
Girlfriend	:	*Hmm...actually I only have one request, but I am not sure whether you can comply or not.*

Man : *Darling, you can mention any requests, diamond, jet plane, big houses, or anything now! What is your request?*

Girlfriend : *Honey, I just want you to sleep eight hours every day for me.*

Man : *Hmm...(sighing and speaking slowly) for that request, I need more time to think about it. You know that I have so many businesses to handle.*

Girlfriend : *But you said you wanted to fulfill all my requests, and now you said you need time to think again...*

Man : *Darling, why do you request such odd thing?*

Girlfriend : *Because I do not want to be alone at my fiftieth or sixtieth. If you really love me, you should not leave me alone when I am old.*

Man : *Okay! (The man is holding his girlfriend's hand.) I promise to sleep for eight hours every day for you. I don't want you to spend your life looking after me in the hospital. We should be together—healthy and enjoying life when we are old.*

An old man sits on a chair in front of his house, closes his eyes, relaxes, and wants to sleep. A young man is passing by the old man house and talks to him:

Young man : *Hi, what are you doing there?*

Old man   : *I am sitting in my chair, relaxing, and wanting to sleep.*

Young man   : *Why don't you use your time to work harder, so you can get a better life and become richer? Don't you have any dreams?*

Old man   : *What for?*

Young man   : *You can buy a big house, car, or other things that are in your dreams.*

Old man   : *After that, what should I do?*

Young man   : *Once you have a big house, car, or other things, then you can relax and sleep.*

Old man   : *So, what do you think I am doing now?*

Young man   : *Hmm..!?@#*

Old man   : *Young man, you don't have to achieve many dreams to relax and sleep well.*

Chapter 15

Frequently Asked Questions

1. *Am I not allowed to take cold water or ice cream?*

   It is better to drink warm water when available, however if you want to drink cold water or eat ice cream, it is recommended that you eat some bread, cookies, a doughnut, or other food first. These foods can absorb some of the cold temperature in your stomach. There are some drinks served at cold temperatures such as iced tea, Coke, honey, and other sweet drinks; you don't have to change it into warm temperature, just eat something first.

2. *Why are we more concerned about water temperature than food temperature for our stomach?*

   Because people usually chew food not water. Water goes directly to our stomach when we drink, but foods are difficult. We need to chew foods, and while chewing, some of the foods' temperature will be absorbed by mouth, teeth, and saliva before the foods go to stomach.

3. *Is room temperature 26° Celsius (78.8° Fahrenheit) a fixed standard?*

This room temperature is a guideline; when you are sick or haven't had enough sleep or in certain conditions, your body may feel cold at this temperature. Then it is okay to adjust the temperature to suit your body; however in normal body condition, setting a room temperature as close as possible to this temperature is recommended. We can also adjust the room temperature when there are many people or electrical equipment installed in that room.

4. *How do I set room temperature at 26° Celsius (78.8° Fahrenheit) when outside temperature is 30° Celsius (86° Fahrenheit)?*

You can set auto AC at 26° Celsius (78.8° Fahrenheit) or you can set manually 4° Celsius below 26° Celsius, which is 22° Celsius to balance the outside weather temperature temporarily. The 4° Celsius is calculated from 30° to 26° = 4° Celsius.

5. *I don't have a water dispenser. What should I do?*

The simple answer is "buy one" or alternatively you can use a hot water container or Thermos to provide warm water when you need it. You can mix the warm water with your drinking water.

It is also a good habit to take a hot water container/Thermos to your bedroom or office, so you can always drink warm water.

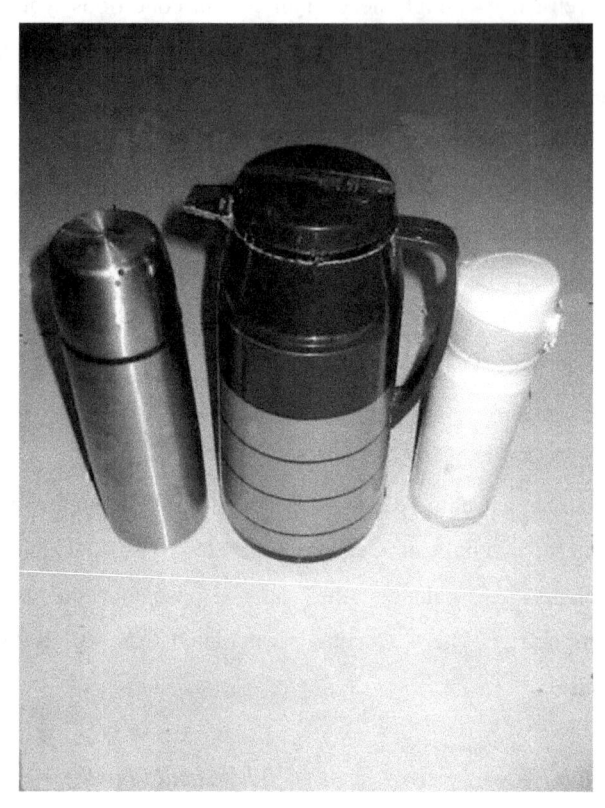

(Hot water containers)

6. *My BMI (body mass index) is in normal range. Should I reduce my meals?*

When you drink warm water and sleep eight hours a day, you can actually reduce your meal portions; however, if you think that your current meals are suitable for your BMI (normal range), and you sleep eight hours a day and drink warm water regularly, you don't have to reduce your meals again. Reducing your meal portions is a trial-and-error process to find a suitable meal size that leaves you within normal BMI standard. At first, you can try reducing meals by one-quarter for one to three months. If you are not satisfied with your resulting BMI, you can reduce current meal portions by only one-eighth.

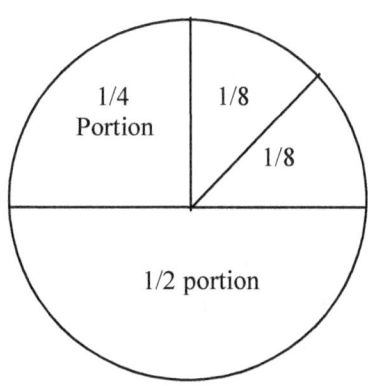

(A portion of food for meal)

7. *Can I change my meal portions when I need more energy?*

    If you think that you have temporary additional activities that are beyond your normal activities, you can return the meal portion to your normal portions (before reduction) temporarily; the point is that you can only reduce you meal portions and not increase the meal portions to exceed your current portion. Your current meal portion is the standard point by which to measure the addition and reduction of your meals.

8. *What if I still feel hungry after reducing my meals and running the system?*

    Try eating more fruit for the additional energy. You can take fruit with you to your office or as you run errands and eat it when you feel hungry.

9. *Can a pregnant woman practice all those recommended exercises?*

    A pregnant woman has a different condition—there are two people in one body. It is better to take a doctor's advice first before following any exercises in this book. It is also recommended that those who are in a sick condition seek a doctor's advice first.

10. *Can I sleep for seven hours or less instead of eight hours?*

    Some people say that you need to sleep for eight hours, and some say seven hours is enough because it depends on the quality of your sleep. But how do you know the quality of your sleep? It is a little bit difficult to have the exact answer on the quality, and that's why there is a recommended range for sleeping time of between seven and eight hours.

Let's calculate the investment you make for sleeping eight hours instead of seven hours. If you are twenty-years-old and you plan to reach 100-years-old, you only need to add around three years [7] investment by changing your sleeping time from seven hours to eight hours. If you are now fifty-years-old, you only need to invest around two years (similar to getting a master's degree) to get a chance of reaching 100- years-old. Of course, it is better to start sleeping eight hours a day habit as soon as possible and not wait until you reach 50- years-old because health is built with daily habits.

What if you sleep for five or six hours a day? This means you invest less than you should, and you may not get the satisfied health return. You may not have enough energy to defend yourself from viruses or bacteria or metabolic problems when they attack you. To illustrate this, you can look at a fighting game on a play station; if the hero does not have enough energy to fight, and he is hit by the enemy several times, he will be knocked out easily by the enemy. The game is over, which means your life is over.

Your body has biological clock, if you usually sleep seven hours, you will wake up after seven hours sleeping; if you usually sleep for five hours, you will wake up after five hours

---

[7] (100 years – 20 years) x 1 hour / 24 hours = 3.33 years

sleeping. So the biological clock is not your standard for the hours of sleeping because if you usually sleep for eight hours, you will also wake up after eight hours of sleep.

In summary, you can sleep for seven or eight hours (or in between) a day to get enough body energy. The additional time investment to reach eight hours of sleep needs to be considered when you have enough time because it only takes around two to three years in your life to add one hour from seven hours sleeping to eight hours sleeping in a day.

11. *Why should we sleep eight hours at night rather than during the day?*

Our eyes do not have night vision, and our ears lack ultrasonic hearing ability; that means we should hide (switch out the light) and sleep at night to protect ourselves from enemies (viruses, bacteria, and metabolism problems). Do you imagine a deer is having fun at night in the moonlit jungle? A lot of enemies (predators) will be watching her, looking for a chance to attack her. These facts indicate that sleeping at night and waking up in the morning is best for us; if you want to wake up at 6:00 A.M., then you should go to sleep at 10:00 P.M. (eight hours of sleep).

12. *If most people drink warm water, will that increase the world energy consumption?*

My simple answer is don't think too much. When you are sick or in hospital, the world does not think about you, and no one feels your pain. Concern about this matter is similar to concern about energy for making coffee or tea.

13. *I am still young and healthy, and currently I do not have any problems that cause sleep debt. What is your opinion?*

Wealth is built penny by penny not by one-night jobs; the same is true of health. Health is built with daily habits not by one-night changes. So, it is better you do not have many sleep debts by paying them as soon as possible because you don't know when they will seize your liver, kidneys, heart, nerves, etc. Having sleep debts also increase the risk for accidents; please don't risk your life when you are young.

14. *Can I use cold water to burn calories and get in better shape?*

There are many ways to burn calories such as running, swimming, and cycling. All these activities increase your health (you use your energy wisely). When you drink cold water to burn calories, it will have a negative impact on your digestive system, and you start the butterfly effect in your body's metabolic process. So, I do not agree with burning calories by drinking cold water because it does not increase your health.

15. *Why do we feel fresher when we drink cold water?*

What do you feel when you go shopping and buy a branded laptop, mobile phone, bags, or dresses? Do you feel fresher? That is because you still have money to buy these things, but what if you don't have money? You may save money for your lunch! Similar to that situation, when we are healthy, we feel fresher by drinking cold water. What if you are sick or have a fever? You may beg for warm water to save your energy. You can have unlimited money in your bank to satisfy your desire, but you cannot have unlimited energy in your body to satisfy your desire. We are in a war situation now, and it is your decision to save your energy or not.

16. *What about pranic or other alternative energy healing?*

Western medical healing methods usually do not pay a lot of attention to this eastern way of healing. There are a lot of arguments from West and East on this healing method, however, as long as it does not have negative effects on your body and you treat this as an addition to your doctor's medical treatment, why not try it?

Every thing in our body is moved by energy, and if there is a person who has talent to heal with energy from his body or the universe or God, we need to appreciate him. Jesus is an example of a person who healed people with his energy (God energy). However, if you are asked to take any herbs or other medicines as part of that alternative healing, you must make sure the practitioner is a professional. It is better that you consult with your doctor first before taking those alternative medicines.

17. What is your comment on a vegetarian diet?

There is nothing wrong with this eating style, however, it should be pure vegetarian. There are some vegetarian restaurants that serve fake chicken, fake pork, fake duck, fake shrimp, etc. to accommodate a vegetarian who wants to eat all these meats. If it is not a matter of religion or a health issue, you are better off eating a little bit chicken, pork, duck, or shrimp than those fake ones. You should ask yourself how those fake meats can manipulate your tongue. A pure vegetarian does not have any intention of eating meat—real or fake. They eat vegetables, fruits, wheat, cereal grains, nuts, etc.

However, don't think that being a vegetarian is a guarantee for longevity; it is just a matter of food composition chosen by a person.

18. Use of food preservatives and flavorings follow government standards, so it should be okay to take them, right?

I do not know how those food preservatives and flavorings are measured in our body. I think the concept is: they measure it in some healthy people and declare those levels of preservatives and food flavorings do not have any negative effect on the human body. What if you only sleep for four or five hours a day and your liver does not have enough rest and may have difficulty handling those preservatives and flavorings? Do the preservatives have any negative effects on your body? In the future, I think all measurements of food preservatives and flavorings should use people who sleep for four hours a day (we are trying to be conservative) and see whether there is a negative impact. This is to make sure that people who even sleep only four hours in a day are okay consuming those preservatives and flavorings.

19. *Will the author be healthier and have longer life than other people?*

The information in this book forms a system. If the author does not follow the system, he can get sick easily and die faster than you.

Appendix

- 0 -

Digestive System

1. Teeth

Teeth chew foods into smaller parts that can be swallowed. There are several enzymes from saliva involved in this digestive process. When time permits, try to chew all your food into smallest parts especially meats (beef, chicken, pork, etc). There is no standard for chewing food but the range of thirty to seventy times is commonly used.

2. Esophagus

The esophagus pushes the foods from mouth into stomach (swallowing).

3. Stomach

Foods are digested in stomach up to four hours; therefore, it is better that you do not eat anything within that four-hour period except fruits because they can be digested easily. There are several digestive enzymes and stomach acid involved in this process. So please try to drink warm water during your meals to save stomach energy and to make sure all the enzymes from your saliva, stomach, pancreas, liver, and intestines are at their best temperature to do their jobs.

4. Pancreas

The digested foods (chyme) are neutralized from an acidic environment by pancreas to allow pancreatic enzymes work.

5. Small Intestine

The digested foods are mainly absorbed in small intestines, and for further processing, they are delivered to the liver by the blood.

6. Liver

There are many functions of the liver and some of them are:
- Monitoring the body energy in the blood
- Cleaning the poisonous materials such as drugs, alcohol, pesticides from the blood
- Breaking down fats
- Storing several vitamins and minerals
- Controlling the body temperature.
- Producing body chemical substances in metabolic process.

After knowing all these liver functions, try not to eat too much meat (beef, pork, chicken, etc.), cheese, milk, oily foods, and fried foods when you have sleep debts because this organ will work harder to break down the fats.

When you take any medicines, please make sure you have enough sleep to help your liver clean the poison from the medicines; otherwise you can get the side effects of the medicines easily and start a new problem for your body. Alcohol should be avoided when you take medicines.

If you are hungry, your stomach is sending a signal to your brain and instructing you to eat something; if you are tired, your liver is sending a signal to your brain and instructing you to sleep or rest. Having coffee or an energy drink when you should sleep or rest is challenging your tired liver to work harder, and this is similar to challenge your hungry stomach with chili. Please do not challenge your liver because you will always lose the game!

Liver is one of the important organs in body metabolism and immune system, so please keep your liver healthy by sleeping for eight hours in a day.

7. Large Intestine

The undigested foods become feces in the large intestines. Having papaya fruit regularly may help solve problems with the large intestine, especially constipation (hard feces).

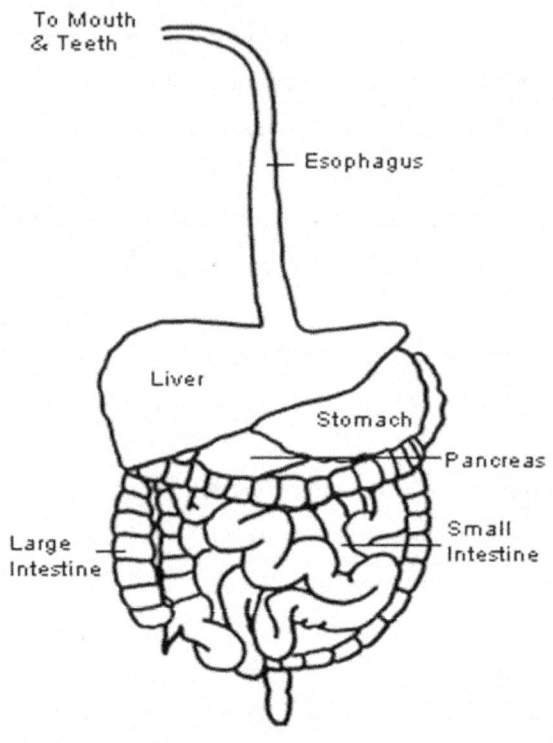

(Human digestive organs)

Oldest man offers diet advice for long life

An article by Sidney George titled "Oldest Man Offers Diet Advice for Long Life" was published at www.greatfallstribune.com as this book was nearing completion. It can give us some knowledge about what he does for his meals.

I would like to say thank you to the writer Sidney George and the *Great Falls Tribune* for giving me permission to quote this article in my book.

Oldest man offers diet advice for long life

September 23, 2009

By SYDNE GEORGE
for the Tribune

So what does the world's oldest man eat? The answer is not much, at least not too much,

Walter Breuning, who turned 113 on Monday, eats just two meals a day and has done so for the past 35 years.

"I think you should push back from the table when you're still hungry," Breuning said.

At 5 foot 8, ("I shrunk a little," he admitted) and 125 pounds, Breuning limits himself to a big breakfast and lunch every day and no supper.

"I have weighed the same for about 35 years," Breuning said. "Well, that's the way it should be."

"You get in the habit of not eating at night, and you realize how good you feel. If you could just tell people not to eat so darn much."

His practice of skipping supper began when he first moved to Great Falls from Minneapolis in 1918. He lived in the Yellowstone Apartments at the time and would walk downtown to Schell's in the Johnson Hotel or the Albon Club on the second floor for lunch.

In 1980, the Albon Club moved to the Rainbow Hotel, and the owners asked Breuning to be manager, which he did for 15 years.

"I never started eating supper again," Breuning said.

He gets up at 6:15 in the morning and has a big breakfast every day at 7:30. Usually it's eggs, toast, or pancakes.

"You can order anything you want, just like a restaurant," he said.

"I eat a lot of fruit every day."

Gov. Brian Schweitzer sent Breuning a fruit basket after a recent visit.

"Boy, I tell you that was good fruit. I ate the whole darn thing," Breuning said. "Peaches, pears, everything. It sure was good."

In addition to eating fruit every day, Breuning also takes a low-dose aspirin.

"Just one baby aspirin," he said, "but everybody gets that for their heart. That's the only pill I ever take—no other medicine."

And he drinks plenty of water.

"I drink water all the time," he said, and just a bit of coffee. "I drink a cup and a half of coffee for breakfast and a cup with lunch."

Breuning said he has been healthy all of his life and believes diet has a lot to do with it.

"If people could cut back on their normal weight, it wouldn't be quite so bad," he commented. "They just eat too much!"

Breuning remembers his family having a cow, pigs, chickens, and a big garden when he was growing up, like most people did in those days.

"Everybody was poor years ago," he said. "When we were kids, we ate what was on the table. Crusts of bread or whatever it was. You ate what they put on your plate, and that's all you got," Bruening said.

Breuning recalls his mother being a good cook, though she died when she was 46 after an operation in Minneapolis. His wife was a good cook, too. They met when they worked in Butte for the railroad.

"Everything she made was good," Breuning said. "We used to have lots of card parties, and they would always say what a good cook she was."

While diet has contributed to his longevity, Breuning also believes that working hard was good for him.

"Work doesn't hurt anybody," he said, mentioning that he had two jobs, one working for the Great Northern Railway until he was 66 and the other as manager/secretary for the local Shriner's Club until he was 99.

These days, Breuning keeps busy talking with all of the people who visit the Rainbow Retirement Center interested in meeting the world's oldest man.

Though his vision doesn't allow him to read anymore, Breuning keeps his mind active by listening to the radio.

"My eyes are gone," he said, "but I listen to the radio. I get all my news on KMON."

Breuning started eating out 35 years ago, but said he doesn't anymore.

"Once you get used to not eating in restaurants, you don't want to anymore," he said. Besides, he'd rather eat at home, the Rainbow Retirement Center.

"They have a lot of good food right here," he said, "and good cooks."

Breuning celebrated his 113th birthday with not one, but two cakes, one chocolate and one vanilla. And for his birthday lunch he got his favorite: liver and onions.

Some notes from author on the article:

Reduce your meals, don't forget to eat fruits, and have a social life/activity when you are old.

Reducing meals without feeling too hungry can be done by controlling the externals and internal environments (see: Chance to live more than 100 years chart – page 88).

References and recommended reading

- 0 -

References and recommended reading

Almatsier, Sunita. _Prinsip Dasar Ilmu Gizi_. Jakarta: Gramedia Pustaka Utama, 2009.

Atkin, Robert C. _Dr. Atkins' New Diet Revolution_. New York: Avon Books, 2002.

Byrne, Rhonda. _The Secret._ New York: Atria Books, 2006.

Carnegie, Dale. _How to Stop Worrying And Start Living_. New York: Pocket Books, 2004.

Clason, George S. _The Richest Man in Babylon_. New York: Signet, 1988.

D'Adamo, Peter J. and Catherine Whitney. _Blood Type O Food Beverage and Supplement Lists_. New York: Berkley, 2002.

Fisher, Philip A. _Common Stocks and Uncommon Profits and Other Writings_.by Philip A. Fisher. New York: John Wiley & Sons, 1996.

Kiyosaki, Robert T. and Sharon L. Lechter. _Rich Dad's Guide to Investing: What the Rich Invest in That the Poor and Middle Class Do Not!_ New York: Warner Books, 2000.

Kiyosaki, Robert T. and Sharon L . Lechter. _Rich Dad's Retire Young Retire Rich: How to Get Rich and Stay Rich Forever_. New York: Warner Books, 2002.

Marsden, Kathryn. *The Complete Book of Food Combining; A New, Easy-to-Use Guide to the Most Successful Diet Ever.* London: Piatkus Book Ltd., 2005.

Naisbitt, John. *Mind Set!* New York: HarperCollins, 2006.

Royston, Angela. *Under the Microscope*: Digesting. Connecticut: Grolier Educational, 1998.

Sherwood, Lauralee. (2006) *Human Physiology: From Cells to Systems.* 6th ed. California: Brooks/Cole, 2006.

Shinya, Hiromi. The Enzyme Factor. Oklahoma: Council Oak Books, 2007.

http://science.education.nih.gov

http://www.cdc.gov

http://www.helpguide.org

http://kidshealth.org/parent/

http://www.who.int

http://health.howstuffworks.com

http://health.yahoo.com

http://www.theclimateprojectus.org